Health Action Zones

Health Action Zones (HAZ) were one of the earliest and most prominent area-based initiatives launched by the New Labour government in England soon after it came to power in 1997. *Health Action Zones*, written by members of the team undertaking the national evaluation of HAZ, examines their development and impact from a variety of perspectives.

The authors outline important features of the social, policy and evaluative environment within which HAZ were established and which greatly contributed to learning about health policy and practice development in the early part of the twenty-first century. They also discuss enduring themes such as building and developing capacity with diverse and unequal partners within complex policy systems. The authors assess the successes of specific strategies aimed at improving health and reducing health inequalities.

Health Action Zones provides in-depth analysis of a key policy initiative that will be of great value to those concerned with building the evidence base for future action. It also offers guidance on how best to design, implement and evaluate future initiatives intended to deal with fundamental social problems.

The multidisciplinary nature of this text makes it suitable for a wide range of postgraduate courses including those covering issues in public health, community care, urban studies, social policy, health and social care research, local governance and public services. The book will also be of great interest to policy-makers and practitioners working in health and community services.

Marian Barnes is Professor and Director of Social Research in the Institute of Applied Social Sciences, University of Birmingham, and Honorary Senior Research Fellow at South Birmingham Mental Health Trust. **Linda Bauld** is Senior Lecturer and Director of the MA in Public Policy in the Department of Urban Studies, University of Glasgow. **Michaela Benzeval** is Research Project Director of the West of Scotland Twenty-07 Study, MRC Social and Public Health Sciences Unit, Glasgow. **Ken Judge** is Head of Public Health and Health Policy and Director of the Health Promotion Policy Unit, in the Faculty of Medicine, University of Glasgow. **Mhairi Mackenzie** is Lecturer in Public Health and Health Policy, in the Faculty of Medicine, University of Glasgow. **Helen Sullivan** is Professor, Urban Governance in the Cities Research Centre, University of the West of England, Bristol.

Health Action Zones

Partnerships for health equity

Marian Barnes, Linda Bauld,
Michaela Benzeval, Ken Judge,
Mhairi Mackenzie and
Helen Sullivan

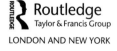

Routledge
Taylor & Francis Group

LONDON AND NEW YORK

First published 2005 by Routledge
2 Park Square, Milton Park, Abingdon, Oxfordshire, OX14 4RN

Simultaneously published in the USA and Canada
By Routledge
270 Madison Avenue, New York, NY 10016

Routledge is an imprint of the Taylor & Francis Group

© 2005 Marian Barnes, Linda Bauld, Michaela Benzeval,
Ken Judge, Mhairi Mackenzie and Helen Sullivan

Typeset in Malaysia by EXPO Holdings, Malaysia
Printed and bound in Great Britain by TJ International Ltd,
Padstow, Cornwall

British Library Cataloguing in Publication Data
A catalogue record for this book is available from the
British Library

Library of Congress Cataloguing in Publication Data
A catalog record for this book has been requested

ISBN 0-415-32551-X (pbk)
ISBN 0-415-32550-1 (hbk)

Contents

Illustrations

Figures

Boxes

Tables

Preface

Like many people in the health community in 1997, we greeted New Labour's election commitment to tackle health inequalities with huge enthusiasm. After so many years of so much research seemingly hitting brick walls, the sense of excitement that things would change for the better was immense. It is hard now, seven years on, to remember the intensity of that feeling, but it is important to try, since this was the world into which Health Action Zones were born.

At the local level the desire to become a HAZ – to be in the 'vanguard of the war on inequalities' – was strong. Being able to talk freely about health inequalities, to discuss the social determinants of health and to think about how to address them represented a radical transformation of the environment in which many local players operated. Every locality wanted to 'lead the way', to be part of the tide of new thinking about how to reduce the health divide.

Equal excitement was apparent in the academic community; a range of new challenges was opening up. No longer was it sufficient simply to find new ways of articulating the problem of health inequalities; instead evidence was required on how to design, implement and evaluate solutions. The tender for the national evaluation of Health Action Zones when it was advertised seemed central to this endeavour. As a result, competition was fierce and bids were ambitious. Ours drew on relatively new theory-based approaches to evaluation, which aimed to find out *how and why* initiatives worked so that effective lessons could be learnt for future polices to reduce health inequalities. When we finally won the bid, the elation at being part of this movement, to have the opportunity to make a difference to the health divide was great, if short-lived. Stakeholders' expectations of what the evaluation could deliver were huge, varied and often conflicting, and the promise of the new approaches to evaluation was much harder to implement in the real world than on paper.

Seven years on, HAZs have been and gone. They and the evaluation did not get the expected chances to deliver real change and learning over the long term. Nevertheless, in their shortened lives there is much that can be learnt from their experiences about how to build on a variety of different foundations in a range of different contexts to develop local capacities for collaboration, for whole systems change and for tackling health inequalities. This book unpacks different aspects of their experiences to examine what can be learnt about how to achieve strategic change locally to build equity in health.

The book falls into three parts. In the first four chapters we set out key dimensions of the changing context of the HAZ initiative and its evaluation. Chapter 1 examines the problems of health inequalities, and what needed to be done to reduce them. Chapter 2 looks at the policy framework, which New Labour introduced, with its emphasis on partnership, participation and place and on developing evidence about 'what works'. Chapter 3 details the approach that was adopted to the evaluation of HAZs within the context of broader thinking about evaluating complex community initiatives. Chapter 4 describes the evolution of HAZs, their broad characteristics and activities, and how they responded to changing policy and political fortunes over time.

The middle part of the book articulates the different stories of HAZs and what can be learnt from them told through a number of different lenses. In Chapter 5, we examine the experience of HAZs in building capacity for collaboration both among statutory agencies and with the community. Chapter 6 considers the extent to which HAZs were able to develop the capacity for whole systems change, while Chapter 7 reflects on what can be learnt from HAZs about how to focus strategies on tackling health inequalities. Finally, Chapter 8, considers local perspectives on HAZ achievements, and the factors that impacted on them.

The last part of the book, Chapter 9, reflects on our experience of undertaking the national evaluation, not only to consider the overall contribution of HAZs, but also to look to the future in terms of what we have learnt about how to evaluate and learn from such initiatives in the future.

The team that has written this book does not include all those who submitted the bid in 1997. In part this is a result of the changes in the size and scope of the evaluation, and in part it is a result of personal changes for different members of the team at various points in time. We would like to take this opportunity to acknowledge the contribution of some of the key people who have worked with us as part of the evaluation team, and from whom we have gained many valuable insights. Our thanks go to Nick Mays, Angela Coulter and Anna Coote, who helped shape the initial bid for the evaluation; to Amanda Killoran, Ray Robinson, Rachel Wigglesworth and Hannah Zeilig, each of whom contributed to the scoping phase of the evaluation; to Louise Lawson, Elizabeth Matka, Fiona Meth, Jane Mackinnon and Julie Truman, researchers on the main part of the evaluation, but who have now moved on to other things; to Sarah Wehner, Teresa Brasier and Martha McCorkindale for all of their organisational skills in keeping us in order at different points on the project. We would also like to thank colleagues in the Department of Health (DH) and National Health Service Executive (NHSE) who supported both HAZs and ourselves in these endeavours. Particular thanks go to Christine McGuire in the DH Policy Research Programme. Most of all, however, we would like to thank the many, many people who have worked in HAZs and given up their time to share their enthusiasm, knowledge and learning from those experiences, so we in turn can share them more broadly.

The national evaluation of HAZs has been a challenging experience. Working in a multidisciplinary team with very differing views on key approaches to the evaluation has made for some lively exchanges along the way. Some of these will be apparent in reading through the different chapters of this book. But through such diversity, we hope that valuable new ways of thinking about the design, implementation and evaluation of local initiatives to tackle health inequalities have emerged. By sharing these in this book, we hope that further learning about building partnerships for equity in health will develop.

This book draws on research undertaken as part of the national evaluation of Health Action Zones, which was funded by the Department of Health. The views expressed in the publication are those of the authors and not necessarily those of the Department of Health. We are grateful to The Stationery Office for permission to reprint a diagram from *Cross-cutting Issues Affecting Local Government* (Stewart et al. 1999).

Marian Barnes (University of Birmingham), Linda Bauld (University of Glasgow), Michaela Benzeval (Queen Mary, University of London), Ken Judge (University of Glasgow), Mhairi Mackenzie (University of Glasgow) and Helen Sullivan (University of the West of England).

April 2004

Abbreviations

ABI	area-based initiative
CCI	comprehensive community-based initiative
CDP	Community Development Project
CHD	coronary heart disease
CYP	children and young people
DETR	Department of Environment, Transport and the Regions
DH	Department of Health
EPA	Education Priority Area
HA	health authority
HAT	Housing Action Trust
HAZ	Health Action Zone
IMD	Index of Multiple Deprivation
LA	local authority
LS	*Longitudinal Study*
LSL	Lambeth, Southwark and Lewisham
LSP	Local Strategic Partnership
MaST	Manchester, Salford and Trafford
NDC	New Deal for Communities
NESS	National Evaluation for Sure Start
NHS	National Health Service
NHSE	National Health Service Executive
NRF	Neighbourhood Renewal Fund
NSF	National Service Framework
PCG	Primary Care Group
PCT	Primary Care Trust
SEU	Social Exclusion Unit
SMR	Standardised Mortality Ratio
SRB	Single Regeneration Budget
ToC	Theory of Change
UDC	Urban Development Corporation

Chapter 1

The legacy of health inequalities

Michaela Benzeval and Ken Judge

Introduction

When New Labour came to power in the United Kingdom in 1997 it brought with it a strong commitment to reducing inequality and social exclusion. Its election victory was greeted with great enthusiasm. Many people believed that comprehensive and purposive public action would make a real difference to the growing social injustices that were evident across all aspects of British life. New Labour itself was determined not to waste the opportunity given to it and quickly introduced a wide range of initiatives to tackle social exclusion and poverty. But it became obsessed with detailed issues of delivery. An excessive reliance on top-down targets, and an ill-placed faith in its own ability to micro-manage complex change processes, perhaps reflected the relative inexperience of ministers during New Labour's first term in office.

Seven years and more on from the landslide election victory that brought the Blair government into power, much of the initial enthusiasm for a centralist approach to 'big' government has waned. But the commitment to promoting social justice remains. What has changed is that there appears to be a more sophisticated recognition of the complexity, pervasiveness and durability of the social problems that have to be confronted. At the same time, there is greater awareness of the need to learn the lessons from past attempts to promote social change. With the benefit of hindsight, many of New Labour's first flurry of social policy initiatives now look naive and over-optimistic. The enthusiasm for evidence-based policy-making, for example, quickly gave way to a desperate scrabble for quick wins to substantiate the 'can-do' rhetoric of the government as it became increasingly clear that the scientific basis for effective interventions to reduce long-standing problems such as health inequalities was remarkably weak. In these circumstances, it would be easy to dismiss the first generation of policy initiatives and to move on, but that would be a mistake and a waste. There is much of value to learn from the early attempts by New Labour to deliver on its election promises. This book seeks to contribute to that process.

One strand of New Labour's initial strategy involved a focus on area-based initiatives (ABIs) to reduce the effects of persistent disadvantage in neighbourhoods blighted by generations of poverty and neglect. Health Action Zones were the first example of this type of intervention, and their focus on community-based initiatives to tackle the wider social determinants of health inequalities excited great interest both nationally and internationally. Like so many other initiatives, HAZs were established in relative haste as high-profile pathfinders that were intended to modernise health care and reduce health inequalities in the most disadvantaged parts of England. One consequence is that they quickly lost their relatively high profile as the policy agenda filled with an ever-expanding list of new initiatives to transform public services and promote social justice. By the beginning of 2003, after most of them had been active for half or less of their intended seven-year lives, they were to all intents and purposes wound up. Nevertheless, the main purposes for which they were established remain important.

So what can be learnt from the experience of Health Action Zones? This book draws on a wealth of findings from the national evaluation of the initiative. It provides a context for and an overview of the HAZ experience, and it explores why many of the great expectations associated with HAZs at their launch failed to materialise. Among the questions it addresses are:

- is there a useful tale to be told about policy failure?
- or is there perhaps a story of progress in the face of adversity?

The answer turns out to be a bit of both. Throughout the book evidence is provided that adds up to the conclusion that HAZs made a good start in difficult circumstances rather than that they failed.

In telling some of the many stories that have to be told to make any sense of the HAZ experience, there are important lessons to be learned about the design, implementation and evaluation of complex community-based initiatives that seek to tackle social problems such as health inequalities. But before our collective impressions of the nature of the HAZ journey and its implications begins, it is important to provide some contextual material about the most important of the issues that they were established to address. To understand both the limitations and the potential of the HAZ initiative, it is essential to have some appreciation of the nature of the problem of health inequalities, the latest scientific evidence about their causes, and the possible role of local action in any strategy to reduce them.

Health inequalities: the problem

Health inequalities have been documented in Britain for over 150 years (Benzeval 2002), and despite considerable increases in overall life expectancy during the twentieth century, they continue to persist to the

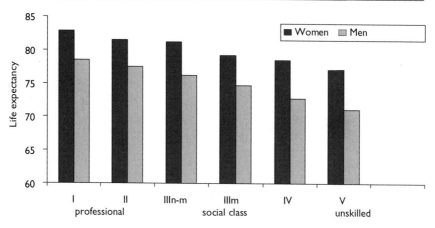

Figure 1.1 Life expectancy at birth by social class, LS, England and Wales, 1997–9
Source: Donkin et al. (2002, Table 1)

present day (Donaldson 2001). However, what is meant by the term 'health inequalities' (Whitehead 1992; Braveman and Gruskin 2003) and how the phenomena are measured (Mackenbach and Kunst 1997; Kawachi et al. 2002) are both the subject of considerable debate. Moreover, there are a number of different dimensions of health inequalities – social, geographic, gender and ethnic – that are considered to be important. There is not room to explore all of the relevant issues here; instead evidence about the main inequalities identified by the Labour government as important policy objectives – geographic and socio-economic (DH 2001b) – is considered. However, most commentators, including the government, recognise that other dimensions of inequalities in health such as those between men and women (Annandale and Hunt 2000) and among different ethnic groups (Nazroo 1999) are important.

Evidence about inequalities in life expectancy at birth among socio-economic groups in the late 1990s is shown in Figure 1.1. Taken from the *Longitudinal Study* (LS), these data show that boys born to professional parents in 1997–9 could expect to live to the age of 78.5, 7.4 years longer than those born to fathers with unskilled occupations. The equivalent gap for girls is 5.7 years.

There are also considerable differences in mortality among different areas of the country. Figure 1.2 shows the Standardised Mortality Ratio (SMR) for different regions within England, and the four countries of the United Kingdom. The whole of Scotland and the North East and the North West of England have SMRs considerably higher than the UK average, whereas the South West and the South East benefit from much lower relative

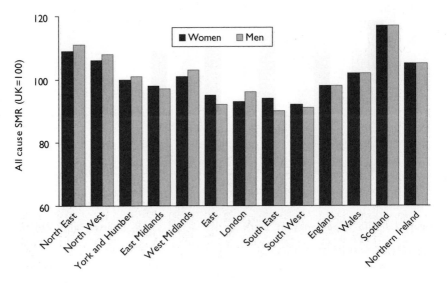

Figure 1.2 All cause Standardised Mortality Ratios by region, UK, 2000
Source: ONS(2002, Table 3.14)

mortality rates. As the Chief Medical Officer commented in his annual report for 2001, such differences are 'not new':

> Throughout the 20th Century, parts of northern England have shown consistently higher mortality than other parts of the country. Despite overall improvements in health, the inequalities gap between socially disadvantaged and affluent sections of the community has widened. A new analysis has shown that some communities in England have death rates equivalent to the national average in the 1950s.
>
> (Donaldson 2001, p. 3)

Donaldson makes two important points that require further exploration. First, he emphasises that such geographic differences are linked to social disadvantage and affluence, and second, that such inequalities are widening.

A wide range of studies has grouped geographic areas by different measures of socio-economic status to show that geographic inequalities in health are the result of socio-economic differences among places. For example, Shaw and colleagues (1999) grouped parliamentary constituencies by their average income to show a very steep health gradient. A revised version of their analysis is shown in Figure 1.3. In 1998/99 parliamentary constituencies with average incomes in the bottom 10 per cent of the distribution had a SMR for under-75s approximately 38 per cent higher than the British average, while those areas in the top 10 per cent of the income distribution had a SMR 20 per cent lower than the average.

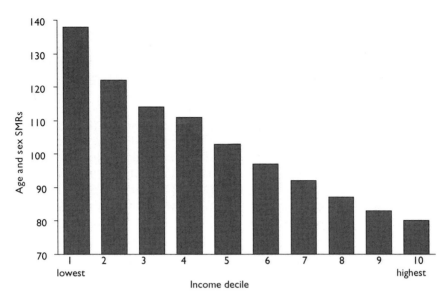

Figure 1.3 SMRs under 75 by parliamentary constituencies grouped by income, Britain, 1998–9
Source: Davey Smith et al. (2002, Table 1)

The same study suggested that inequalities in health among parliamentary constituencies had widened during the 1990s (Davey Smith et al. 2002), while other studies have showed a widening of inequalities between areas in the 1980s (e.g. Phillimore et al. 1994) and within regions in the 1980s and 1990s (e.g. Reid and Harding 2000). Similarly, at the individual level, studies have shown widening inequalities between social classes since the 1970s based on a range of measures of health and socio-economic status (Drever and Whitehead 1997; Hattersley 1999). On the other hand, a few studies have suggested that there may have been a narrowing of inequalities at the end of the 1990s. For example, Whitehead and Drever (1999) found evidence of a reduction in social inequalities in health for infant mortality, and Strong and colleagues (2002) found a narrowing of geographic inequalities in mortality within Trent region. Other studies, however, have found that the way in which inequalities are measured over time can affect whether or not trends appear to be widening or narrowing (Donkin et al. 2002; Rees et al. 2003).

Health status and socio-economic circumstances are difficult concepts to define and measure, and the ways in which this is done can affect the estimate of the size of the problem (Manor et al. 1997; Macintyre et al. 2003). The composition and size of social groups varies over time, and whether or not these factors are considered may affect comparisons over time (Benzeval et al. 1995a). Similarly, whether relative or absolute differences in health are considered, whether differences between two groups (i.e. the most affluent and the most disadvantaged) or across the whole population are compared, and whether simple or sophisticated measurement techniques are employed, will also affect the scale of inequalities estimated from any particular dataset (Mackenbach and Kunst 1997) and hence whether or not they appear to be increasing or decreasing over time.

Despite these measurement difficulties, there is overwhelming evidence about the existence of social inequalities in health across the developed world, with a number of countries beginning to develop strategies to address them (Mackenbach and Bakker 2002). In England, the government has also acknowledged that health inequality is a substantial and persistent problem that needs to be addressed (DH 2003c). The next section, therefore, considers the causes of health inequalities and the general kinds of policy solutions advocated to reduce them.

The causes of health inequalities

A significant landmark event in the study of health inequalities was the publication in 1980 of the *Black Report* (Townsend and Davidson 1982), an independent inquiry commissioned by the Callaghan government in 1977. The report suggested that the four most likely explanations for social inequalities in health were that they are:

- an artefact of measurement error
- the product of social selection
- caused by individuals' behaviours
- a result of individuals' material and social circumstances.

After carefully reviewing all of the evidence available at that time, the inquiry concluded that the materialist explanation was the most significant cause of health inequalities, although each of the others also made a minor contribution.

Since the publication of the *Black Report*, a huge research endeavour has been conducted to explore and assess the relative importance of these different explanations further (Macintyre 1997a; Graham 2000b). In general, this evidence, which has been based on increasingly sophisticated datasets and analyses, supports the broad findings of the *Black Report*. However, these explanations are not without their critics and a number of extremely acrimonious debates have developed between academics exploring different kinds of arguments in relation to them (Macintyre 1997a).

Nevertheless, when the second independent inquiry into health inequalities, commissioned by the New Labour government in 1997, reported in 1998 it came to a similar conclusion to that of the *Black Report*.

The weight of scientific evidence supports a socioeconomic explanation of health inequalities. This traces the roots of ill health to such determinants as income, education and employment as well as to material environment and lifestyle.

(Acheson 1998, p. xi)

Such assessments have been accepted by the government and form the foundation of its strategy to address health inequalities (DH and HM Treasury 2002; DH 2003c), as discussed in Chapter 2. However, such a succinct summary of causation belies the complexity of the underlying relationships and pathways, and hence the difficulties of designing policies to reduce inequalities in health. As Graham (2000b) points out:

A single pathway would, of course, simplify the explanatory task and provide a 'clear' steer to policy makers seeking to reduce health inequalities. However, the evidence points to multiple chains of risk, running from the broader social structure through living and working conditions to health related habits like cigarette smoking and exercise. ... The chains of risk have been uncovered primarily through surveys of individuals. However, a small seam of research is beginning to locate individuals in the places in which they live and to suggest that both individual factors and area influences have their part to play.

(Graham 2000b, p. 14)

This is not the place to discuss the mass of evidence that explores the different explanations for health inequalities in depth. (For a more in-depth discussion of these issues see the collection of evidence submitted to the Acheson Inquiry (Gordon et al. 1999) or the summary of the findings of the Economic and Social Research Council (ESRC) research programme on health inequalities (Graham 2000a).) However, the key message is that health inequalities are the result of an individual's social and economic circumstances across their life course. An important corollary is that a key determinant of health inequalities is the general social and economic inequalities that exist in England at the present time (DH 1998d).

England has experienced considerable social and economic change in the last few decades. A reduction in manufacturing industry and a growth in the service sector has led to a reduction in male employment, particularly among unskilled workers, and a growth in mainly female, often part-time, employment (Graham 2000b). This, together with the increasing number of lone-parent families over the same period, led to a growth in the number of working-age households where no one was in paid employment. By the second half of the 1990s, such families accounted for one-fifth of all working-age households (DH 1999b).

These trends, together with changes in benefit and taxation policies implemented by Conservative governments in the 1980s (Goodman and Webb 1994), contributed to a massive increase in the number of families living on low incomes and consequently a dramatic growth in income inequality, of an almost unprecedented degree compared with other industrial countries (Atkinson et al. 1995). By 1998/99, 14.3 million people (about one-quarter of the population) and 4.4 million children (approximately one in three) lived in households with less than half the average income (Gordon et al. 2000).

Alongside these economic trends there has also been considerable social change. The rise in the number of lone parents has already been mentioned; over 3 million children, one-quarter of all families, live in one-parent households. There has also been a dramatic rise in owner occupation of houses, which has led to the marginalisation of social housing that is increasingly restricted to the most disadvantaged sections of the community. For example, around two-thirds of heads of households in social housing are unemployed, compared with about one-third in other housing tenures (Rahman et al. 2000).

Together the labour and housing market changes exacerbated geographical inequalities in poverty and wealth in England (Graham 2000a). Overall, the 1980s and 1990s experienced significant increases in unemployment, people living on low incomes, lone-parent families and social and geographical polarisation (Benzeval 2002).

Against this background, most commentators have argued for the need for a range of reforms to national social and economic policies to address health inequalities (e.g. Townsend and Davidson 1982; Benzeval et al. 1995b; Acheson 1998; Shaw et al. 1999). Policies advocated include: increasing income support, reducing child poverty, promoting employment and education, improving the availability of affordable housing, and making health care more equitable. The extent to which New Labour have taken these ideas on board in their evolving strategy to address health inequalities is discussed in Chapter 2. However, one of the first policies introduced by New Labour in relation to health inequalities was a specific local initiative – Health Action Zones. The next section examines what they were and how they were expected to tackle health inequalities.

The HAZ initiative

The newly elected Blair government announced its intention to establish HAZs in June 1997. The aim was to:

> explore mechanisms for breaking through current organisational boundaries to tackle inequalities, and deliver better services and better

health care, building upon and encouraging co-operation across the NHS.

(Dobson 1997)

The proposed establishment of HAZs was the first ABI announced by New Labour and the only one led by the Department of Health.

Following the initial announcement, a support team for the initiative was established within the NHS Executive (NHSE) in Leeds. Its remit was to develop policy in relation to HAZs and to organise a bidding process for HAZ status. Health authorities (HAs) were invited, along with partners such as local government and the voluntary sector, to submit bids in October 1997. The bidding guidance set out the government's aspirations for HAZs in relation to health inequalities:

> HAZ status will provide added impetus to the task of tackling ill-health and reducing inequalities in health ... HAZ status will be long term, spanning a period of five to seven years, recognising the need for strategic change. There will, however, need to be evidence of change taking place and of concrete gains for local people throughout that period.
>
> (DH 1997a, para 3)

More specifically the guidance set out three strategic objectives for the initiative:

- to identify and address the public health needs of the local area
- to increase the effectiveness, efficiency and responsiveness of services
- to develop partnerships for improving people's health and relevant services, adding value through creating synergy between the work of different agencies.

The guidance made it clear that in order to tackle health inequalities, bids were expected from areas 'of pronounced deprivation and poor health'. Forty-nine bids were received from forty-one HAs. The Secretary of State for Health played an active role in the selection of the successful bidders. They were chosen for a range of reasons connected to particular legacies of industrial decline and poor health or specific health issues, as well for their development plans for tackling health inequalities (Milburn 1997). At the end of the process eleven areas were selected to become first wave HAZs, and were officially launched in April 1998 (DH 1998b). The bidding process for the second wave HAZs was more restricted, with invitations to bid sent to only thirty-four HAs in the most deprived areas. An objective tool for assessing the bids was developed by the HAZ team in the NHSE. Recommendations were made to ministers on the basis of the strength of the bid against the set criteria, although how closely this was followed is open to question. A further fifteen HAZs were selected and launched in April 1999 (DH 1998c).

In general, there was considerable criticism of the selection process. For example, Powell and Moon (2001) argued that the specific criteria for the selection of HAZs were never clearly articulated, making it difficult to understand the rationale behind the initiative. Others, focusing on government claims that HAZs were from the most deprived areas, questioned this and pointed out that bids from more deprived areas had been rejected (Shaw et al. 1999). Finally, a number of commentators highlighted the political interference that had taken place in relation to the HAZ bids both in terms of the geographic areas that they covered and the priorities they established (Painter with Clarence 2001). There is some truth in these and related concerns but this should not obscure the fact that many parts of most HAZs were among the most deprived neighbourhoods in England.

The HAZs

Box 1.1 shows the location of the twenty-six HAZs. They were located in diverse areas of England, although mainly concentrated in the North and the Midlands, with only four Zones in London, one in the Home Counties and two in the South West. The HAZs varied considerably in their population size and organisational configurations. While some HAZs were based on partnerships between one health authority and one local authority, others had much more complex structures. The resulting geographical coverage of individual HAZs was both an enabling and a disabling feature of their endeavours (Benzeval 2003a).

HAZs were given dual roles in relation to reducing health inequalities. First, they were meant to improve health outcomes and to reduce health inequalities in their areas.

> Health Action Zones are a key part of the Government's drive to target areas with particularly high levels of ill health ... and so improve the health of the worst off at a faster rate than the general population. This is the first time a British Government has set itself such a task.
>
> (DH 1998c)

Second, HAZs were expected to act as 'trailblazers' and to take the lead in developing new ways of tackling local health inequalities.

> Health Action Zones are in the vanguard of our new approach to tackling health inequalities and promoting new ways of working together locally between health and social services.
>
> (Denham 1999)

Box 1.1 Health Action Zones

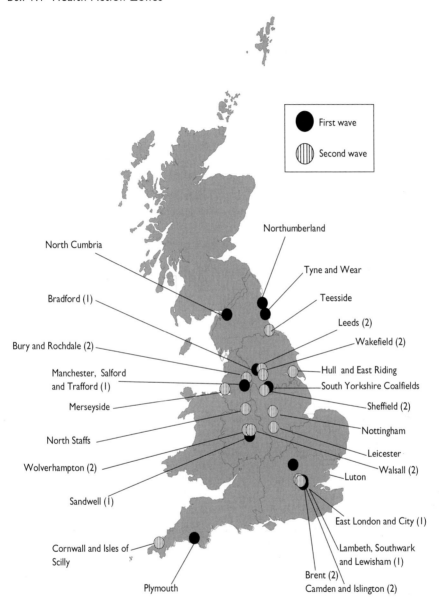

Health Action Zones are in the frontline of the Government war on health inequalities. They have both the opportunity and the responsibility to pioneer new ways of driving up local standards of health.

(Jowell 1999)

In establishing HAZs, the DH explicitly recognised the importance of addressing the wider determinants of ill health. As a result HAZs were expected to invest in activities that would help to 'join up' services that affect the root causes of ill health such as employment, education, housing and poverty. In order to achieve this, effective partnerships had to be developed at the local level. In practice HAZs built upon the partnerships they had formed to submit their bids and established multi-agency boards to coordinate the initiative at the local level. These boards were confronted with an ambitious set of expectations articulated by central government. These included modernising and reshaping services, engaging communities, setting targets for their programmes of work, and developing performance management systems that would act as a tool through which agreed milestones and targets could be monitored (Judge et al. 1999).

As 'pioneers' and 'trailblazers' in tackling health inequalities, HAZs had not only to invest in innovative initiatives and ways of working but also to establish effective ways of learning from them. They were expected both to mainstream successes internally and to disseminate good practice more broadly to the health community.

The Department of Health provided HAZs with modest resources – for example, the initial allocation of £320 million over three years (1998/99 to 2001/02) represented less than 1 per cent of NHS funds in HAZ areas (Judge et al. 1999). HAZs were also promised longer term funding of up to seven years. They received some money for development support, totalling approximately £100,000 per year per HAZ, which was used primarily to pay the salary of a project manager (who was responsible for the day-to-day running of the HAZ), modest administrative support and costs associated with maintaining the partnership board(s) that would provide strategic direction for the HAZ. In addition to these resources, HAZs were provided with additional resources earmarked for specific purposes, related to smoking cessation services, pump-priming drug prevention programmes, innovation projects, employment and health projects and the establishment of Healthy Living Centres.

The initial response to HAZs

From the outset, while there was considerable enthusiasm for the HAZ idea among practitioners, significant questions were raised by a number of academics about whether or not HAZs were an appropriate vehicle for tackling health inequalities. The key focus of such concerns was that local action could not address the structural causes of social and economic problems and hence health inequalities.

Although there has been a long tradition of investigating geographic differences in health, it was not until the early 1990s that researchers began to ask whether such variations were simply the result of the socio-demographic composition of the population that lived in the different areas or whether there were important 'area', 'place' or 'contextual' effects on health (Macintyre et al. 2002). Partly driven by the availability of new large datasets and increasingly sophisticated analytical techniques, much of the initial work in this field concentrated on trying to unravel statistically the relative importance for health of compositional (the characteristics of people that make up an area) and contextual (the characteristics of places themselves) effects (e.g. Sloggett and Joshi 1994; Duncan et al. 1996; Shouls et al. 1996; Wiggins et al. 1998). Overall, this research suggests that most of the differences in health among areas are the result of compositional effects, although 'area characteristics' play a small part.

As a result of these kinds of findings, a range of commentators have argued that tackling poverty nationally is the best way of tackling health inequalities locally (e.g. Sloggett and Joshi 1994; Mitchell et al. 2000a). Such commentators argue that the underlying structural causes of health inequalities, such as unemployment and poverty, can be addressed only through national policies to promote employment and to improve incomes through the tax and benefit systems (Shaw et al. 1999). Similar arguments are made about regional policies and ABIs more generally (e.g. Massey 2001). It is clearly true that major reductions in poverty require such fiscal reforms, and should in time reduce health inequalities (Benzeval et al. 2000). 'Inequalities in health are a national problem that require national solutions' (Shaw et al. 1999, p. 177). However, it does not necessarily follow from this that local investment across the range of complex determinants of health cannot contribute to reducing the health divide. While it requires national changes in policy to increase benefit levels, for example, local initiatives can be very effective in ensuring greater uptake of such benefits in ways that improve the incomes of the worst off (e.g. Hoskins and Smith 2002).

Another argument critical of the creation of HAZs, and ABIs more generally, was that most 'poor people' do not live in 'poor areas' (Shaw et al. 1999). Targeting areas in order to reduce the poverty experienced by individuals, therefore, is bound to fail. However, Powell and colleagues (2001a) argue that as well as tackling 'people poverty', governments also need to address 'place poverty', i.e. areas with inadequate services in different policy domains, and that the two do not necessarily overlap in the same geographical space. If 'place poverty' is regarded as a significant feature of British society, then ABIs, including HAZs, may have been an appropriate policy response. More generally, there is increasing recognition in the health inequalities literature of the importance of a range of local factors in the causal chain of health inequalities.

The role of local factors in determining health inequalities

Much of the existing academic work investigating the relative importance of the characteristics of people and the characteristics of places for individual's health has been criticised for the lack of theoretical basis in conceptualising how places might affect health (Mitchell et al. 2000b; Macintyre et al. 2002), and for falsely dichotomising the two effects (Macintyre et al. 2002; Curtis 2004). Macintyre (1997b) argues that there is a third explanation for geographic differences in health that should be considered – the collective properties of local people. This suggests that sharing socio-cultural histories with other people who live in the neighbourhood may influence people's health (Macintyre et al. 2002). For example, the concentration of particular ethnic groups in a community may influence the facilities available in the local community, such as the types of food and shops, leisure and entertainment facilities; the shared norms of the community in terms of health beliefs and practices; and, an individual's sense of belonging and identity (Curtis 2004). All of these factors may influence people's health.

In reality, therefore, it is the interaction of the characteristics of people with local social and economic structures that is likely to influence people's health (Popay et al. 1998, 2003; Curtis 2004). There have been a number of attempts to conceptualise how the characteristics of places might affect health. For example, Curtis (2004), drawing on a range of social theories, suggests that places may have different conceptual landscapes that will affect people's health.

- *Ecological landscapes* include aspects of the physical environment, such as pollution and other hazards, which may affect the local population's health. Exposure to environmental hazards such as air pollution is likely to be higher in areas occupied by disadvantaged communities than wealthier areas (Curtis 2004).
- *Consumption landscapes* refer to the availability of local goods and services, which will affect individuals' access to key resources for health such as healthy food, health care facilities, etc. For example, there has been increasing concern that certain disadvantaged areas of Britain may be 'food deserts', i.e. have little local access to shops selling nutritious food at affordable prices (Curtis 2004). Similarly, within health care, there is concern about the operation of an 'inverse care law', i.e. that areas with the most need have the least services (Tudor Hart 1971).
- *Landscapes of poverty and wealth* include factors such as local economic conditions, which will impact on an individual's own social and economic circumstances in ways that affect their health. For example, conditions in the local labour market will influence whether or not an individual can find a job; the kinds of positions available to them; and, hence their living standards and their health.
- *Landscapes of power* relates to the ways in which the power structures that individuals encounter in their everyday lives may affect their health. There is a particular focus on the ways in which less powerful groups in society may be excluded or marginalised in ways that damage their

health. For example, travellers, refugees and people who are homeless often find it difficult to access the services and resources that they need for their health, and are stigmatised by the wider community in ways that further exclude them (Curtis 2004).

- *Therapeutic landscapes* draw on ideas from cultural geography about the positive effects of the 'sense of place' on health (Gesler 1992). Traditionally such research focused on 'healing places' such as Lourdes or Bath Spa, but is increasingly being used to investigate the effect of other spaces on health, for example, the natural environment in general, as well as the home and health care facilities (Curtis 2004).

More specifically, for example, researchers at the Medical Research Council (MRC) Social and Public Health Sciences Unit, at the University of Glasgow, have undertaken a range of different studies that have directly tried to examine specific features of local areas and the ways in which they may be health enhancing or health damaging. In such work they identify five types of features (Macintyre et al. 2002):

- physical features of the environment shared by all local residents
- availability of healthy environments at home, work and play
- services provided to support people in their daily lives
- socio-cultural features of a neighbourhood
- the reputation of an area.

The last two of these categories relate to the social functioning and practices of an area; ideas closely related to the notion of 'social capital' (Macintyre et al. 2002), which has been explored in considerable depth in the public health literature (e.g. Cooper et al. 1999; Swann and Morgan 2002). Social capital is typically seen as a contextual or environmental construct, part of the societal structure of an area, encompassing formal and informal social connections as well as norms of reciprocity and trust (Subramanian et al. 2003). As such it is a complex concept, which has been measured in a wide variety of ways in different studies (Curtis 2004). Moreover, there has been strong criticism in the literature about the lack of theoretical underpinning and construction of the concept itself (MacKian 2002), and of the ways in which it may improve health (Veenstra and Lomas 1999).

A number of quantitative studies have demonstrated an association between living in areas of 'high social capital' and an individual's health (e.g. Kawachi et al. 1997). However, other studies suggest that the influence of socio-economic factors is much more important than that of social capital (Cooper et al. 1999). There is some evidence that social capital may act as a buffer between some of the effects of neighbourhood poverty on health (Cattell 2001). Other commentators have argued that the assumption that social capital is a 'good thing' for communities and that it can be operationalised to invigorate 'unhealthy' communities is open to question. The promotion of social capital among some groups in society may benefit those particular groups but to the detriment of others (MacKian 2002).

Nevertheless, a range of commentators have argued that local action to promote social capital may be an important way of addressing health inequalities. For example, Gilles (1998) argues that the most successful health promotion initiatives focus on the needs of communities rather than individuals, and utilise and promote social capital to improve health. Whether this is a valid assumption or not, such ideas were influential and initiatives to promote social capital were an important feature of the work of Health Action Zones, as discussed later in this book.

We do not want to suggest that local initiatives are likely to solve the problem of health inequalities on their own. In common with many other commentators we believe that effective action to reduce virtually all manifestations of social inequalities requires fundamental changes to national policies in areas such as tax and benefits, education and enterprise renewal. But at the same time we also think that local initiatives have a useful contribution to make to address manifestations of problems that vary from place to place. Local partnerships can contribute to tackling health inequalities by responding to variations in needs and values, testing and refining new ideas, contributing to the evidence base and simply demonstrating possibilities. Health Action Zones attempted to do many of these things. A careful review of their experiences, therefore, ought to strengthen future attempts to improve health and reduce inequalities. The remainder of this book sets out to do just that.

Chapter 2

Public policy under New Labour

Marian Barnes, Helen Sullivan, Michaela Benzeval, Ken Judge and Mhairi Mackenzie

Introduction

New Labour came to power in 1997 with an ambition to transform public policy and public services. Central to the achievement of this ambition was the development of 'joined-up government' within Whitehall as well as across central and local government. The government embarked upon a variety of strategies in order to facilitate this. Some critical assessment has questioned the extent to which these strategies actually constituted a consistent approach to a single shared concept of 'joined-up government' (Ling 2002). However, what can be deduced from the discussions and debates in both the policy and academic spheres is a clear intent to transform public policy and public services and to do this by adopting a different perspective on governing and by looking at policy problems in what were claimed to be new and different ways (6 P 1997; Richards et al. 1999; Stewart et al. 1999; Sullivan and Stewart 2002). This chapter will examine the key characteristics of the New Labour approach to public policy, and locate the HAZ initiative within this context. It will address the drivers for 'joined-up government', consider how policy developed to address the health inequalities documented in Chapter 1, discuss the '3 Ps', partnership, participation and place, which characterised much New Labour policy, and refer briefly to the concept of 'evidence-based policy-making', claimed to underpin the whole approach.

'Joined-up government'

Upon taking office in 1997 New Labour was faced with a public policy system that was fragmented and ineffective in service delivery. It was also a system that had experienced significant reform at the hands of previous Conservative administrations. In 1979 the public policy system had still been characterised by features which were introduced in the 1940s, including the organisation of government around functional spending departments, the operation of hierarchical modes of management and decision-making, the privileging of professionals and professional judgement in service decisions and the clear separation of central and local government and their remits. The Conservatives sought to challenge various aspects of this system, including curbing the power of professionals through the strengthening of a managerial culture and the introduction of market 'disciplines' to public services (Clarke and Newman 1997). The rationale for this was couched both in terms of the belief that individuals and families should take responsibility for themselves and not become 'dependent' on the state, and also within a consumerist discourse which emphasised the right of consumers to choose both the nature of the services they used and who provided them. While this did not result in a significant shift from public to private health care provision, there was an important expansion in the private provision of social care services, and within both health and social care agencies there were substantial changes to the organisation of services which were intended to separate out service delivery from responsibility for service purchasing or commissioning (LeGrand and Bartlett 1993; Barnes 1997a).

The consequences of such a radical programme of reform across the public policy system were to vastly increase the number of different kinds of service delivery agents, including 'in-house' providers, quangos and private sector bodies; to pose new challenges for the securing of accountability in an environment where the traditional mode of governing through hierarchy had been diminished by the introduction of markets and networks; and to blur the boundaries between central and local, for example by introducing new delivery mechanisms that operated locally but were accountable centrally (Stewart and Stoker 1995; Ferlie et al. 1996). In different ways these developments acted to fragment the operation of government and the development and delivery of public policy. For New Labour the task was to make the system work effectively without returning to a 1940s-style public policy system. The government recognised and indeed supported an accommodation of market principles, service user choice and the operation of networks in a process of 'modernisation' of public services and public policy-making.

The challenges to New Labour's 'joining-up' endeavour arose not just from the actions of prior administrations. Another development – multi-level governance – played an important role in changing the prevailing governance environment and challenging the capacity of the central state to secure a less fragmented future. Multilevel governance has been defined as

> negotiated, non-hierarchical exchanges between institutions at the transnational, national, regional and local levels ... [which] do have to operate through intermediary levels but can take place directly between, say the transnational and regional levels, thus bypassing the state level.
>
> (Peters and Pierre 2001, p. 132)

The evolution of multilevel governance may have acted to loosen the taut central–local relationships in the United Kingdom by providing opportunities for localities, sub-regions and regions to operate beyond the central state. Evidence of this is provided via examples of global–local relationships exemplified by Local Agenda 21 environmental programmes, Healthy Cities and *Health For All* initiatives, and European Union (EU) – regional/local relationships manifest in the Committee of the Regions established following the Maastricht Treaty of 1991.

Nevertheless, the UK central state has retained considerable influence in shaping the development of multilevel governance, most obviously through the establishment of new institutions such as the Scottish Parliament and Assemblies in Wales and Northern Ireland. However, through the devolution programmes of the 1990s including the creation of 'Next Step' Executive Agencies (such as the Benefits Agency) and local quangos to deliver a variety of local services (such as Training and Enterprise Councils), the state also precipitated the need for horizontal relationships to be developed to mobilise resources and overcome fragmentation.

In association with its developing approach to governing, New Labour also sought to rethink its understanding of policy problems. The post-war welfare state had been designed around the 'five giants' which Beveridge had identified as standing in the way of post-war development: want, disease, ignorance, squalor and idleness (Timmins 1995). A failure to solve these problems through various manifestations of the state led some observers to the view that this was not merely an organisational problem, rather it was also the way in which 'problems' had been separately delineated. The concept of the 'wicked issues' (Rittel and Webber, 1973) was advanced to refer to core policy problems which could not be addressed by any one agency because the problems themselves could not be separated one from another – the issue of health inequalities is an obvious example. For Clarke and Stewart (1997) addressing 'wicked issues' required holistic rather than linear thinking, capacity to operate outside conventional organisational, professional and assumptive boundaries, and the involvement of the public in finding solutions to these problems. In such circumstances the role of government was to 'enable' or 'orchestrate' action rather than exercise direct control of implementation (Rhodes 1997; 6 P et al. 1999).

Elsewhere in Europe the concept of 'social exclusion' was being advanced to capture the multidimensional nature and impact of the experiences of those most affected by the 'wicked issues' – those marginalised from mainstream society (Berghman 1995). The 'problem' of social exclusion was seen to have many dimensions and tackling it successfully required attention to be paid to each of these dimensions in a coherent and co-ordinated way with an emphasis on outcomes rather than inputs or process of service delivery. This reconceptualisation of the nature of policy problems has been significant in the development of what is arguably leading to a more profound transformation of the public policy system under New Labour than that resulting from the consumerist and market-driven ideology of the previous Conservative governments. Barnes and Prior (2000) identify three aspects of this which characterise most of the public policy initiatives taken by the New Labour government, which display a commitment to the ambition of 'joined-up government' and which were embodied within the HAZ initiative – at least within its aspirations:

- A change in focus from a service delivery to an issue and locality-based approach. The appeal to 'partnership' between the various agencies of the state and beyond as a means of developing shared solutions to the interconnected policy problems was central to the new approach and required 'joined-up' working at all levels from neighbourhood to Whitehall.
- The balance shifted from a highly individualised notion of a public service consumer, to an emphasis on people as members of communities. 'Relationships between individuals and communities are conceived as sources of identity … a source through which people can both receive welfare and, perhaps more importantly, create the conditions for their own well-being' (Barnes and Prior 2000, p. 96). In this way public participation can enhance the development of 'joined-up government'.
- Related to both of the above – communities were identified not only as the place within which problems are located and solutions must be found, but also as the sources of many of those solutions. This brings us back to the first point: the partnerships through which solutions will be found and delivered will include not only statutory agencies and those within the private and formal independent sectors, but also community organisations, user groups and individual community members.

From 'variation' to 'inequality' in health

The issue of health inequalities can be considered a prime example of a 'wicked issue'. Chapter 1 documented the massive accumulation of evidence on health inequalities and some of the key debates about their causes. However, throughout most of the tenure of the 1979–97 Conservative government, action to tackle them was noticeable mainly by its absence (Benzeval 1997). It was not until 1995 that a specific report focusing on 'health variations' was published (DH 1995). While the Conservative government was not prepared to use the language of 'inequality', this report did represent a significant change in the government's approach. At long last, the existence of 'social variations in health' was explicitly acknowledged by the Department of Health and a policy response, albeit limited to the NHS, put forward (Benzeval 1997). At the same time the *priority and planning guidance for the NHS* began to identify 'reducing variations in health' as a policy issue (NHSE 1996).

Despite the negative national policy context during this period, some, if not all, health authorities had developed initiatives to improve the health of disadvantaged communities or to increase access to health care in deprived areas (Benzeval 1999). In addition, from the mid-1980s onwards, many HAs adopted the *Health For All* targets and/or became healthy cities (Laughlin and Black 1995), both of which have reducing inequalities in health as a central component of their aims (Ashton and Seymour 1988). However, such initiatives were often at the margins of HAs' activities, and evaluations over this period found that they had not been incorporated into mainstream planning or priorities in any systematic way (Rathwell 1992; Goumans and Springett 1997).

More broadly, a number of reviews attempted to assess and document HA action in relation to health inequalities. In the main, these reviews came to the same, rather negative, conclusions (see e.g. Dearden 1985; Castle and Jacobson 1988; Laughlin and Black 1995). Taken together, the evidence suggests that by the late 1990s, and as the change of government approached, few local agencies had much experience or knowledge about how to establish strategic partnerships to tackle inequalities in health locally. The HAZ initiative was the first concerted government strategy to address health inequalities. But it was not the only policy through which the government sought to address this problem.

Broader policies to address health inequalities

At the same time as HAZs were initially launched, the New Labour government also began to develop its strategy to tackle health inequalities more broadly. One of the aims of this strategy was 'to improve the health of the worst off in society and to narrow the health gap'. It acknowledged the social causes of ill health and inequalities and noted that 'tackling inequalities generally is the best means of tackling health inequalities in particular' (DH 1998d, p. 12). It identified a range of policies that were being implemented to reduce poverty and social exclusion as evidence of progress in this respect.

To support the development of its strategy, the government established the Acheson Inquiry to review the evidence base for attacking health inequalities. This set the framework for subsequent policy discussion of population health and health inequalities in England. The Acheson Report made three key recommendations:

- All policies likely to have an impact on health should be evaluated in terms of their impact on health inequalities.
- A high priority should be given to the health of families with children.

- Further steps should be taken to reduce income inequalities and improve the living standards of the poor.

The government's response to Acheson was set out in *Reducing Health Inequalities: An Action Report* (DH 1999c). This publication 'set out the action that was being taken **across government** – and through partnerships between the various local and regional organisations in England' (p. 3, original emphasis) – that would range across almost all aspects of economic and social policy as part of the commitment to building a fairer society. At the local level, Health Action Zones were highlighted as 'leading the way' (p. 14). The overall programme was claimed to be the most comprehensive programme of work to tackle health inequalities ever undertaken in England. However, it was acknowledged that developing programmes of action and having an impact on health inequalities would take considerable time.

In the three years following the publication of the action report in July 1999, a steady stream of policy announcements related to public health and inequalities was published, although the prominence of Health Action Zones in these statements diminished over time. (See Benzeval 2003, Appendix 1 for an annotated list of key policy statements.) Significant among these policy developments was the announcement of two health inequalities targets focusing on life expectancy and infant mortality. The government's objective was 'by 2010 to reduce inequalities in health outcomes by 10 per cent as measured by infant mortality and life expectancy at birth' (DH 2003c, p. 7), underpinned by two more detailed objectives:

- Starting with children under 1 year, by 2010 to reduce by at least 10 per cent the gap in mortality between routine and manual groups and the population as a whole.
- Starting with local authorities, by 2010 to reduce by at least 10 per cent the gap between the one-fifth of areas with the lowest life expectancy at birth and the population as a whole.

Soon after the two national health inequalities targets were originally set in 2001, the government established an interdepartmental group chaired by HM Treasury to conduct a cross-cutting review to assess progress on health inequalities and to formulate priorities for the future. For the first time it:

> brought together Ministers and officials from across Government departments and from local government, along with academic experts, to consider how better to match existing resources to health need and to develop a long-term strategy to narrow the health gap.
>
> (DH and HM Treasury 2002, p. 2)

A successful endeavour?

The achievements of the early policy programme of the New Labour government in relation to health inequalities are the subject of much debate. The government (unsurprisingly) took a rather upbeat view of its performance. Numerous examples of the progress that was being made were cited in official documentation, including:

- between 1995 and 2000 breastfeeding among low-income groups rose from 50 to 59 per cent
- between 1998/99 and 2001/02 the number of children living in low-income households fell by 400,000
- the number of homes in the public and social housing sectors falling below minimum standards was reduced from 2.3 million to 1.6 million between 1996 and 2001.

However, not all of the presented examples represented prima facie evidence of a reduction in inequalities. For example, the claim that 120,000 people quit smoking at the four-week stage after receiving cessation services says nothing about the social distribution of these beneficiaries. On the other hand there did appear to be evidence of a reduction in road deaths, particularly among children in low-income groups (DH 2003c, paras 3.27, 3.29).

A more independent assessment of the progress made by the government in responding to the recommendations of the Acheson Report can be found in a Joseph Rowntree Foundation report (Exworthy et al. 2003). This study 'identified five dimensions that characterise the progress made and the work that remains'. They are:

- activity related to tackling health inequalities
- policy-making developments across government
- systems to support policies
- embedding policies within structure and processes
- measuring and monitoring progress.

(Exworthy et al. 2003, p. 46)

The authors most readily identified achievements in process terms but concluded that hard evidence of substantial progress in reducing indicators of inequalities was virtually non-existent. However, the report was a positive one and broadly supportive of the government's own position. It concluded that 'many challenges remain but the prospects for tackling health inequalities are good' (Exworthy et al. 2003, p. 52).

If there is one single area of social life that must change, as a prerequisite for closing the health divide, it is to bring about a significant reduction in the extent of poverty, which grew dramatically across the United Kingdom after the mid-1980s. Poverty has a particularly deleterious effect on children, where the number living in low-income households tripled between 1979 and the end of the century when it embraced about one-third of the total, depending on the definition of poverty employed (Sutherland et al. 2003). The New Labour government made clear its commitment to reducing child poverty,

> The Government is committed to reducing by a quarter the number of children in low-income households by 2004–05 (from a baseline of 1998–99) as a contribution towards the broader target of halving child poverty by 2010 and eradicating it by 2020.
>
> (DH 2003c, p. 20)

A study commissioned by the Joseph Rowntree Foundation attempted to assess the government's progress in relation to this target by focusing on two issues (Sutherland et al. 2003, p. 7):

- How and why has poverty in Britain changed?
- How is it likely to change as a result of changes in benefits, direct taxes and indirect taxes?

Obtaining answers to these deceptively simple questions, however, is fiendishly difficult and they depend on very important judgements about underlying assumptions and key definitions. Nevertheless, Sutherland and colleagues (2003) reported some important conclusions including that child poverty was reducing. However, they also concluded that even if the government were to achieve its 2010 target to reduce child poverty by one-half, 'relative poverty will still be higher than in 1979' (p. 63). Moreover, although much attention and success has focused on families and children there are many other groups who have been relatively neglected, and the goal of security for those who cannot work 'is a long way from being achieved' (p. 63).

Developing the strategy

Action to address health inequalities requires a long-term commitment. In July 2003, the Department of Health published its long awaited three-year plan, *Tackling Health Inequalities: A Programme for Action*, which set out an ambitious agenda covering all national, regional and local agencies across England (DH 2003c). The strategy drew on learning from a range of policy initiatives aimed at reducing health inequalities developed in New Labour's first term to consolidate its approach to reducing health inequalities in a more systematic way. It explicitly recognised the need to give priority:

> to tackle the causes and consequences of health inequalities as a part of its commitment to deliver economic prosperity and social justice.

Action to break the cycle of deprivation and its impact on avoidable ill health is at the heart of government policy.

(DH 2003c, p. 9)

The programme made explicit a number of assumptions about those areas of government policy that were likely to have the greatest impact on inequalities over the longer term. It also highlighted key interventions expected to help achieve the main health inequality targets with respect to life expectancy and infant mortality. The programme was organised around four key themes:

- supporting families, mothers and children
- engaging communities and individuals
- preventing illness and providing effective treatment and care
- addressing the underlying determinants of health.

Each of these themes was underpinned by five key principles: preventing health inequalities worsening; working through the mainstream; targeting specific interventions; supporting action from the centre and through the regions; and delivering at the local level. There was a working assumption that solid progress would be made by 2010 but it was also acknowledged that longer term reductions in health inequalities would take a generation or more to achieve and the programme pointed towards 2030 as a useful focal point.

While the HAZ initiative was clearly intended to be one way of addressing the wicked issue of health inequalities, it was also shaped by more general themes characterising public policy under New Labour. These other major themes and their relevance to the HAZ initiative are discussed under the headings of partnership, participation and place.

Partnership

Partnership has become inescapably interlinked with the New Labour project. Almost all significant public policy proposals introduced since 1997 have, to a greater or lesser extent, required the forming of partnerships to secure the desired outcomes (see e.g. Glendinning et al. 2002). Partnership has been at the heart of New Labour's redefinition of relationships between central and local government, with the re-establishment in 1997 (after twenty years in abeyance) of the 'Central–Local Partnership', a forum where key representatives of central and local government seek to improve the way in which the two levels work together.

Partnership has also been key to the New Labour approach to addressing 'wicked issues'. Not only was the Health Action Zone initiative predicated upon health authorities working together with others to create strategic partnerships to identify and address health inequalities, but also the Crime and Disorder Act 1998 required local authorities and the police service to jointly lead local multi-agency Crime and Disorder Partnerships for their areas; the National Strategy for Neighbourhood Renewal (Social Exclusion Unit (SEU) 2001) set out a framework for tackling social exclusion through cross-sector partnerships involving local communities, and government introduced Local Strategic Partnerships (LSPs) to facilitate more efficient and effective targeting of the range of available resources into localities (Department of Environment, Transport and the Regions (DETR) 2000d).

Partnership is also evident in New Labour's programme of public service reform. It features in the creation of 'zone' status for the delivery of improvement in relation to education and employment services as well as health; and in the introduction of public–private partnerships and the Private Finance Initiative to deliver bespoke services and capital projects in key areas, such as health, education and the prison service. New organisational forms such as Health and Social Care Trusts and Children's Trusts bring key public services providers together to offer alternative ways of delivering some of their services.

Of course, partnership working is not new but what is new is the sheer scope and scale of partnership action initiated since 1997. According to Sullivan and Skelcher (2002) 5500 local or regional level partnerships were recorded in the United Kingdom in 2001 that were stimulated or created by government. The authors identified at least sixty different types of public policy partnership from government data, excluding partnerships that might be operating in agriculture and rural development, defence and through European programmes, and partnerships that had been established voluntarily. They also estimate that in 2001/02 between £15 billion and £20 billion was being spent on sub-national partnership activity. While this amount is relatively small in comparison with the totality of the public sector budget, it is significant because of its impact in redirecting mainstream activity towards partnership-supported policy outcomes. Partnership working is also significant for the human resources it consumes: an estimated 75,000 partnership board places at the sub-national level in the United Kingdom in 2001/02 in comparison with 23,000 elected councillors and 60,000 quango places (Sullivan and Skelcher 2002).

From 'coordination' to partnership

The specific interest of central government in trying to secure more effective 'joining-up' between health and social care predates New Labour and can be traced back to the late 1960s. Sullivan and Skelcher (2002) identify three phases in the relationship between health and social care.

- *Developing co-ordination:* in the late 1960s and early 1970s the emphasis was on the co-ordination of policy development and implementation at national and local levels. The application of rationality in public policy was in the ascendancy and co-ordination was perceived to be the most sensible response to 'the complex, untidy sprawl of social boundaries and responsibilities and to the problem of resource scarcity' experienced in health and social care services (Challis et al. 1988, p. 2). This approach was exemplified in the publication of *A Joint Approach to Social Policies* (Department of Health and Social Security (DHSS) 1975) with a core assumption that cooperation would replace competition between ministers of state and their central departments.

- *The mixed economy of care:* this phase began in the early 1980s and focused on broadening the range of providers of relevant services while at the same time acknowledging the continuing need for a co-ordination role. Market mechanisms were introduced into health and social care organisations and an 'internal market' created in health. The NHS and Community Care Act 1990 set out the government's aspirations for the delivery of health and social care services in an integrated way to 'enable people to achieve maximum independence and control over their own lives' (DH 1989, p. 9). Local authority social services departments were given the lead role in managing the community care system. However, the government was criticised for attempting to 'impose' collaboration and partnership working between sectors from the top rather than helping to create the conditions where it might flourish (Hadley and Clough 1996).

- *Supporting strategic collaboration:* New Labour attempted to chart a pragmatic course in relation to 'joining-up' health and social care services, retaining an attachment to rationality and to markets but overlaying this with a strategic service delivery framework, intended to facilitate partnership working between local stakeholders. This strategic framework included the passing of the Health Act 1999 which placed a statutory duty of partnership on the NHS and local authorities, removed some of the legal obstacles to joint working between them and made available a new partnership grant. From April 2000, pooled budgets, lead commissioning and integrated service provision became options that NHS–local government partnerships could make use of. Evidence from a survey of local authorities (Local Government Association 2000) suggested that this supportive approach had a positive impact with 88 per cent of respondents making use of the Health Act flexibilities or planning to do so and almost nine out of ten respondents indicating that the relationships between health and local government had improved since 1997.

Notwithstanding all of this activity and the regularity with which the word 'partnership' was being used (some might say overused), it is very difficult to pin down precisely what New Labour meant by partnership. One explanation for this may be found in a study that preceded the New Labour administrations but which displayed considerable prescience in its assessment of attempts to define partnership. According to Roberts and colleagues (1995)

> Partnership means many things to many people. Indeed it is not clearly defined precisely because its ambiguity can be politically attractive. It is difficult to be opposed to partnerships ... There is no single easily transferable model of partnership.
>
> (Roberts et al. 1995, p. 7)

These reflections alert us not only to the slipperiness of definitions but also to another danger associated with partnerships, the assumption that they are inherently benign rather than neutral instruments, which may be shaped by those who act from positive and negative motivations. One aspect of the assumed 'benign' nature of partnerships is that those involved share equality of power. Experience suggests otherwise and this is one aspect of the HAZ experience that is explored in Chapter 5.

Drawing on the work of those who have studied partnerships in operation it is possible to identify a number of imperatives that drive partnership formation (for example, MacKintosh 1992; Huxham 1996; Hughes et al. 1998; Hudson et al. 1999; Savas 2000). These include achieving a shared vision; maximising the use of available resources; addressing complexity in public policy or service delivery; maximising power and influence; and using partnerships to resolve conflict. Most partnerships will be underpinned by more than one of these imperatives, which may be prioritised differently by different partners, and they will be important in determining the shape and nature of the partnership that develops. The language of the Department of Health's invitation to bid for HAZ status revealed a perspective on HAZs as vehicles for designing and delivering a shared multi-stakeholder vision in relation to improving health and reducing health inequalities. For example, HAZs would 'harness the dynamism of local people and organisations to achieve change' and their creation would 'release local energy and innovation' (DH 1997a). However, it was also possible to identify a concern with using HAZ status and the partnerships associated with this to find alternative ways of tackling the apparently intractable problems associated with complex issues such as health and social care service delivery.

While definitions of partnership may prove elusive, Sullivan and Skelcher (2002, pp. 5–7) elaborate a series of features that one might associate with partnerships in the UK public policy system and which can be applied to HAZ.

- Partnership involves the mobilization of a coalition of interests from more than one domain. HAZs typify this by drawing together stakeholders from the public, private, voluntary and community sectors.

- Partnership involves negotiation between diverse agencies committed to working together. A key assumption made about HAZs was that the initiative would be 'pushing at an open door', that is government was responding to demands that had been made of it by local agents anxious for the opportunity to work across boundaries to address health inequalities and health improvements. For some HAZs this was complicated by the fact that the area granted HAZ status was larger than originally envisaged and brought together a number of health and local authorities that had not previously demonstrated a wish to work together and whose relationships had to be worked out as part of the HAZ programme.
- Partnership aims to secure the delivery of benefits (or added value) which could not have been provided by any single agency acting alone. The government's decision to go ahead with HAZs was in part a recognition of 'health' as a 'wicked issue'. This had long been recognised in many localities where HAZ status provided the legitimacy to pursue the 'value added'.
- The achievements of the partnership are subject to assessment. HAZs, like most New Labour policy initiatives after them, were required to undertake their own local evaluations of progress and were also part of a wider national evaluation of the policy initiative as a whole. This formed part of the New Labour commitment to generating 'evidence-based practice' (see p. 38) but is also associated with the operation of good practice in partnerships (Hudson et al. 1999).

While these features might be common across public policy partnerships, such partnerships can be distinguished in other ways. So, for example partnerships at the local level can be strategic, sectoral (concerned with a specific issue or service) and/or neighbourhood focused. Among the factors that distinguished partnerships of these different types was the extent to which they involved the public in their activities (Sullivan and Skelcher, 2002, p. 167). But while the form and intensity of citizen engagement may vary, what was non-negotiable in much of New Labour's policy programme is the level of attachment to the engagement of the public in initiatives like HAZ. The rationale for this and the experiences of the public in relation to health services is explored below.

Participation

A clear expression of New Labour's belief in the positive agency of communities is evident in this quote from a Social Exclusion Unit publication:

> The most powerful resource in turning around neighbourhoods should be the community itself. Community involvement can take many forms:

formal volunteering; helping a neighbour; taking part in a community organisation. It can have the triple benefit of getting things done that need to be done, fostering community links and building the skills, self-esteem and networks of those who give their time.

(Social Exclusion Unit 1998, p. 68, para 5.26)

The moral imperative implied in the use of the word 'should' in the first line is even more explicit in the conclusion to the same report. In acknowledging the testing goals that the government had set itself in addressing social exclusion, the report identified the responsibilities of government, business and the voluntary sector in achieving these goals. But such responsibilities also rest with citizens: 'they require a willingness on the part of people living in poor neighbourhoods to take up new opportunities' (Social Exclusion Unit 1998, p. 79).

Community involvement is not an option – either for agencies wishing to take advantage of funding and development opportunities associated with new policy initiatives or for members of the communities on which those initiatives are targeted. Both parties have to be prepared to shoulder the responsibilities for action and to work together to achieve change.

There were antecedents for this commitment to engaging citizens in the process of policy-making and service delivery. In the late 1960s and early 1970s there were calls for more effective means of involving the public in local authority planning processes (Hampton 1990). The establishment of Community Health Councils in 1974, for example, was intended to ensure the 'public interest' was represented when major changes were proposed to health services. Community Development Projects marked a brief and marginally effective focus for community involvement in the process of improving local service delivery (Cockburn 1977). This sense of a collective 'public' or 'community' with a legitimate part to play in policy-making and implementation was abandoned during the 1980s and early 1990s in favour of an appeal to individual consumers to exercise choice in a public service market place in order to impact on the quality and responsiveness of public services (Barnes and Prior 1995). But even during the long years of Conservative supremacy, pockets of a more collective approach to user and public involvement were developing and, in some instances, being supported by local authorities, the NHS and other public organisations (Beresford and Croft 1993; Deakin and Wright 1990).

Alongside and interacting with officially sponsored user involvement, public participation and community involvement initiatives, the 1980s and 1990s also saw the growth of collective action on the part of service users, community and identity groups which was in part focused on autonomous 'community building' by groups who experienced themselves as marginalised and oppressed, and in part taking advantage of the spaces that had opened up within the policy process to claim a voice in policy-making (e.g.

Campbell and Oliver 1996; Ledwith 1997; Barnes 1999a; Barnes and Bowl 2001).

The New Labour commitment to community involvement built on this history as well as introducing its own moral and ideological dimension to the type of initiatives it sought to promote. In doing so government ministers were responding to what they perceived as the failures of public services both in terms of governance and service delivery, the weakening of civil society with a resultant loss of 'social capital', and failures of citizens to engage in the democratic practices necessary to a healthy and inclusive society. Prime Minister Tony Blair expressed his personal belief in the importance of 'people' rather than government in achieving a healthy economy and society:

> We have always said that human capital is at the core of the new economy. But increasingly it is also social capital that matters too – the capacity to get things done, to cooperate, the magic ingredient that makes all the difference. Too often in the past government programmes damaged social capital – sending in the experts but ignoring community organisations, investing in bricks and mortar but not in people. In the future we need to invest in social capital as surely as we invest in skills and buildings.
>
> (Speech to National Council for Voluntary Organisations 1999)

Thus, UK public policy when the Health Action Zone initiative was launched prioritised the direct involvement of citizens, both individually and collectively, as a means of achieving better public services; increasing the legitimacy of decision-making; revitalising democracy; creating responsible citizens; and resolving major policy problems. Among the different purposes being advanced for increasing the participation of 'the public' in policy-making, it is possible to identify a number of themes:

- a concern about the nature of public services and their capacity to be responsive to the needs and aspirations of an increasingly sophisticated, knowledgeable and diverse population of 'consumers'
- a questioning of the authority traditionally attached to professionals or other 'experts' and an awareness of the significance of lay and experiential knowledge in decision-making both about individual service use and in shaping public policy
- the interconnectedness of policy 'problems' (the 'wicked issues') and the need to understand how these impact on people's lives as a whole
- a concern that traditional models of representative democracy are losing their legitimacy and failing to engage with sufficient number of citizens.

(Barnes 2002, pp. 166–7)

In practice this led to a diverse and growing number of examples of user, community and public participation in a diverse range of policy and institutional contexts. In a review of participation initiatives in two English cities, Barnes and colleagues (2002) found that motivations for public participation derived not only from national government imperatives – predating New Labour as in the case of the Single Regeneration Budget and Best Value, and post New Labour in the case of e.g. New Deal for Communities (NDC) and Sure Start – but also from supra-national institutions. For example, the European Social Fund was the source of grants for a family support strategy at neighbourhood level in which parents and children were active participants, while the Local Agenda 21 initiative deriving from the Rio de Janeiro environmental summit was the inspiration for a local sustainability forum. There were examples of participation initiatives based in both communities of locality (usually neighbourhoods) and communities of identity, including Senior Citizens Forums, a gay and lesbian forum and Black and minority ethnic communities. Some participation initiatives were based around use of particular services, in particular social and health services, and others around issues, such as poverty or environmental concerns. Others were explicitly focused on renewing democratic practice and sought to introduce direct participation into local representative systems of democracy through the establishment of neighbourhood forums in which local residents could meet with both officials and elected members. Some initiatives also included a specific commitment to building collective capacity among specific communities (Sullivan et al. 2004).

User and public participation in the NHS

Within the context of the development of user and public participation in the NHS it is possible to identify particular characteristics of the way in which health service managers and professionals responded to this imperative (Barnes 1997b). The NHS came rather later than did local government to the view that service users and citizens should have a voice in determining health and health services policy, and service design and delivery. Factors that affected such developments in the NHS context have been identified as follows:

- a loss of or reduced public confidence in individual health 'experts' and in the NHS as a whole in the wake of attempts to introduce market principles
- more readily available information about health, illness and treatment via the internet which has created more knowledgeable and confident consumers of health services
- technological advances (such as in the field of genetics) which have generated questions that cannot be left to science to answer, but demand ethical, moral and political debate

Box 2.1 The development of user and public participation in the NHS

- The NHS and Community Care Act 1990 introduced the internal market and encouraged consumer choice.
- *Local Voices* (NHSE 1992) encouraged HAs to seek public views on health needs and priorities.
- The *Patient's Charter* (1992) introduced procedural rights for individual health service consumers.
- The launch of the *Patient Partnership Strategy* and the establishment of the Standing Advisory Group on Consumer Involvement in the NHS Research and Development Programme in 1996.
- Proposals that the new PCGs should have clear arrangements for public involvement (DH 1997c).
- Developments in both the Patient Partnership Strategy and the R&D Programme during 1998/99.
- The requirement for user and public involvement as a condition for HAZ status.
- Developments emanating from the *NHS Plan* (DH 2000c) and the consultation document *Involving Patients and the Public in Health Care* published in 2001 (DH 2001e): Patient Advice and Liaison Services (PALS) in all Trusts, Patient and Public Involvement Forums in all trusts and PCTs, the coordination of these forums by the Commission for Patient and Public Involvement in Health, established in January 2003.

- the need to maintain public support for the service at a time when radical change was deemed to be necessary
- the persistence and deepening of health inequalities and the need for public involvement to address these
- increased public awareness of health issues and their links to other public policies – such as environmental and food policies.

(from Barnes 1999b)

These factors contributed to a rapidly expanding series of initiatives during the 1990s and early 2000s through which user involvement and public participation became official policy within the NHS. The main 'official' initiatives during this period are set out in Box 2.1.

Alongside these national initiatives were a plethora of local initiatives focusing on service users (from patient participation groups in primary care, to user councils in secure psychiatric hospitals), on geographical communities, and on particular population groups.

The summary in Box 2.1 demonstrates that when the HAZ initiative was launched, there had been important progress within the NHS supporting the development of user and public participation. HAZ itself was seen as a means of prioritising and increasing capacity to this end. However, during the lifetime of HAZ participation became official policy and HAZs were no longer singled out as locations in which one would expect to see participation being prioritised. Nevertheless, in spite of a policy commitment to participation there continued to be reluctance in some quarters. The command structure of the NHS is not sufficient to overcome the resistances identified in reports such as *In the Public Interest* (NHSE et al. 1998) and a change in policy does not immediately generate the skills and attitudes necessary to the new ways of working that user and public involvement requires. The freedoms and flexibilities that it was intended HAZs should enjoy should have enabled them to make a significant contribution to ensuring that involvement and participation went beyond being simply another task to perform.

Among the range of purposes advanced for involving communities in the design and implementation of policy initiatives was that of reducing social exclusion. It has been argued that one dimension of social exclusion is exclusion from those processes through which decisions are taken which have a direct impact on a person's life (e.g. Young 2000). But it is questionable whether the explosion in opportunities for people to take part in debate about policy-making and service delivery has had a dramatic impact on outcomes within the sphere of health and other policy areas. Evaluations of specific user involvement and participation initiatives have pointed to intrinsic benefits accruing to those who take part and to some limited direct effects on services (e.g. Barnes and Bennet 1997). But service users and community members who have had lengthy experience of being researched, consulted and involved in policy processes have also expressed weariness and cynicism about the lack of significant change which has flowed from this. The Barnes et al. (2002) study offered some explanation for this from a detailed analysis of the way in which exchange takes places within participative forums and the consequent potential for the development of alternative and more inclusive discourses (Sullivan et al. 2003b; Barnes et al. 2004). Other detailed studies have similarly suggested that institutionalised ways of thinking and practising can be hard to shift, particularly in situations where the power imbalance is weighted strongly in favour of professionals and other officials (e.g. Ellis 1993; Church 1996). Thus when Health Action Zones were created, it remained to be proved that community involvement had the capacity to achieve the considerable structural transformations that the aspirational authors of the HAZ project were seeking.

'Place'

The third overarching characteristic of New Labour's approach to policy-making has been an emphasis on localities as both a focus and target for interventions. In the history of UK regeneration policy since the mid-1970s, 'place' has always occupied a contested position. There remains an ongoing debate about the extent to which targeting public resources at deprived areas (however specified) will have a greater impact on the population of those areas than channelling resources via mainstream services (Robson et al. 1994; Bradford and Robson 1995). This debate is played out in both policy-making and academic arenas and regeneration policy fluctuates depending upon which perspective is in the ascendancy.

The focus on spatial targeting first emerged in the Education Priority Areas (EPAs) and Community Development Projects (CDPs) of the 1970s. These programmes emerged following an assessment of persistent inequality in urban areas which highlighted lack of co-ordination between public agencies rather than individual pathology as a core source of the problem. EPAs and CDPs were designed to channel additional resources into specified areas and to act to better co-ordinate the application of these with relevant mainstream resources. These partnerships between central and local government were also the basis for subsequent place-based urban policy. Following the publication of the 1977 White Paper, the Inner City Partnership Programme was established. This programme sought to develop a cross-sector partnership in each designated local authority area in order to target additional resources at initiatives in inner city areas. In reality, while voluntary sector bodies benefited by gaining access to funding, neither they nor the private sector were permitted to challenge the core central–local governmental relationship (Barnekov et al. 1990).

While the Conservative regimes of the 1980s and 1990s adopted a very different perspective on regeneration, emphasising the role of the private sector and the channelling of funds through single-purpose agencies (quangos) as opposed to local government, the focus on 'place' did not disappear. In the 1980s Urban Development Corporations (UDCs), powerful local quangos dominated by private sector interests and with a primary focus on physical regeneration, were set up to revitalise specific areas within cities. These were followed by Estate Action programmes designed to diversify the funding and management of social housing schemes at estate level and Inner City Task Forces to improve enterprise and employability among populations in targeted areas of disadvantage.

In the 1990s the focus on 'place' as neighbourhood increased with the emergence of the City Challenge initiative, a neighbourhood-based physical, social and economic regeneration programme. This was followed by the establishment of Housing Action Trusts (HATs) in six localities, single-purpose bodies governed by a board appointed by the Secretary of State. Like City Challenge, the purpose of HATs was the physical, social and economic regeneration of the targeted neighbourhoods with a clear emphasis upon increasing the mixed economy of provision in housing.

The plethora of area-based programmes in the 1980s was subject to criticism in an Audit Commission review which described the emergent urban policy as a 'patchwork quilt of complexity and idiosyncrasy' (Audit Commission 1989, p. 9) and recommended greater co-ordination of activity with an emphasis on strategic intervention and improvement across localities rather than focusing on specific neighbourhoods within them. Consequently a number of changes were made to the way in which urban policy for England was delivered (mechanisms for coordination in Scotland and Wales already existed). Central Government Offices for the Regions were established to co-ordinate activity centrally and to help 'join up' Whitehall departments to improve their interface with localities. In addition a new comprehensive regeneration programme, the Single Regeneration Budget (SRB), was introduced. This programme brought together a range of existing spending programmes into a single pot in order to maximise resource flexibility and offered a role for thematic as well as 'place based' regeneration activities. SRB was one of the longer lasting government initiatives with six rounds of bidding for funds between 1994 and 2000, generating over 900 local partnerships.

According to Sullivan and Skelcher (2002) three main changes occurred in regeneration policy following New Labour's taking office in 1997:

- *The demise of competition:* competing with other localities for funds was largely replaced by targeted spending on key areas based upon indices of deprivation, for example through the Neighbourhood Renewal Fund (NRF), which allocated resources to the eighty-eight local authorities with the highest levels of deprivation. Competition did not disappear entirely. The experience of HAZs illustrates how localities had to make a case for being awarded HAZ status in competition with other areas.
- *Communities in the lead:* partnerships *with* communities gave way to the idea of partnerships *led* by communities, as in the NDC initiative which prioritised the capacity building of community leaders as members of neighbourhood partnerships prior to any decision-making about spending NDC resources.
- *A focus on 'joining-up' key policy priorities:* regeneration policy focused on the synthesising of action in key policy areas – namely education and employment, health, crime and the physical environment. This was initiated in NDC but expanded under the National Strategy for Neighbourhood Renewal so that 'joining-up' occurs within neighbourhoods and also across localities. This would be facilitated through the establishment of a LSP.

So many 'place-based' initiatives were developed under New Labour that they were given their own collective term, area-based initiatives (ABIs). The range of these initiatives also went far beyond the scope of previous regeneration programmes, embracing all manner of policy areas for example:

- *Coalfields programme:* regeneration of coalfields areas.
- *Community Chests:* support community involvement in deprived areas.
- *Creative partnerships:* creative experiences for school children in deprived areas.
- *Education Action Zones:* raise educational standards in groups of schools.
- *Neighbourhood Management:* local integration of services.
- *Sport Action Zones:* bring benefit of sports to deprived areas.

HAZs were one of the first ABIs established by New Labour on taking office and their focus on 'place' was rather more flexible than that of subsequent programmes such as NDCs, which targeted neighbourhoods of approximately 11,000 people. HAZs could be focused on a particular town or city, such as Bradford, they could bring together adjacent districts with shared health concerns, for instance Lambeth, Southwark and Lewisham, they could also acknowledge and address the specific problems posed by 'place', such as the challenge of rural areas like Cornwall and Northumberland as well as the demands of diverse neighbourhoods in urban conurbations such as Manchester. The diversity of the size and coverage of the twenty-six HAZs suggested geography as an enabling rather than constraining feature of the initiative, one which allowed for the adoption of other foci including the targeting of communities of identity or interest across administrative or other boundaries.

In a study of a selection of ABIs undertaken for central government, Stewart et al. (2002) found limited impact of ABIs upon mainstream functions and services and little evidence that individual ABIs had been able to combine their efforts in localities where several ABIs were in operation. Stewart et al. (2002) also identified some 'confusion' in the concept of ABIs, particularly in relation to the differential significance attached to 'place'. They conclude that:

> [o]nly in some ABIs is the area the focus for attention, and there is a distinction between initiatives which happen in areas but are basically functional and initiatives which have the regeneration of the areas at their heart ... The challenge of the neighbourhood-based approach is to make closer linkages between the functional perspective of service planning and delivery and the spatial perspective of neighbourhood renewal
> (Stewart et al. 2002, p. 127)

This reference to neighourhoods points to New Labour's real focus of attention in relation to the issue of 'place'. The UK government's

Neighbourhood Renewal Strategy specified that action to tackle social exclusion needed to be 'joined-up', in order to tackle its multifaceted nature effectively. The related Policy Action Team (PAT 17) report on *Joining it up Locally* (Social Exclusion Unit 2000; Stewart et al. 2002) identified a lack of 'joined-up' action at all levels of government as one of eight reasons why regeneration policies had consistently failed to deliver sustainable improvement in the poorest areas. The report highlighted the significance of 'place', i.e. neighbourhoods as an important site for action but emphasised the need to 'join-up' vertically as well as horizontally in order to achieve sustainable change. It also drew attention to the potential contribution of the public to the tackling of 'wicked issues' like social exclusion, highlighting the need to empower and involve local communities in regeneration programmes. These features are evident in New Labour's commitment to programmes such as the NRF, neighbourhood management, NDC and Sure Start. The rationale for these initiatives reflects that articulated thirty years previously, that is the need to ensure better co-ordination of local services and resources to alleviate poverty and inequality.

HAZs thus occupy a rather ambiguous position in the context of the targeted 'place-based' ABIs promoted by New Labour. Many covered huge areas – in terms of both geography and population – and brought together widely varied places with which few could identify. But much of the work that they undertook *was* targeted within specific localities where it was important to establish good links with local populations and initiatives sponsored by other ABIs. Implicitly, HAZs were understood to offer the advantages both of co-ordination across areas that were linked by geographical proximity and social problems experienced, but separated by administrative authority; and of targeted locality or neighbourhood based action. In common with similar initiatives which aim to address social problems through targeted rather than universal action, they were based on an assumption that it is possible to identify particular places in which customised initiatives will 'work' to relieve structural inequalities.

Evidence-based policy-making

The final characteristic of public policy-making under New Labour that needs attention here is the emphasis on 'evidence-based policy-making'. The evaluation on which much of this book is based was an expression of this commitment. Policy is required to be 'implemented (or sustained) on the basis of strong supporting evidence that the policy will (or does) work' (Oliver and McDaid 2002, p. 183). Policy evaluation is thus seen as an integral part of evidence-based policy (Oliver and McDaid 2002). The New Labour government claimed: 'what counts is what works' (Davies et al. 1999, p. 3) and evaluation became a core feature of the design of social programmes (Nutley and Webb 2000; Solesbury 2001). Broad issues concerning the nature and impact of evidence-based policy-making are discussed elsewhere (see for example Davies et al. 2000a; Nutley et al. 2003). There are also substantial critiques of many of the assumptions underpinning this approach, including the way in which notions of 'evidence' are constructed (e.g. Harrison 1998; Fischer 2003; Yanow 2003). Two interrelated issues relevant to shaping evaluation within an evidence-based policy context are highlighted here: evidence about the ways in which evaluations are utilised in the policy process, and the effect of commissioning evaluations within an evidence-based policy context on the scope, conduct and expectations of the evaluation.

Rational models of policy-making assume policies develop in a linear fashion. First, a problem is identified, second, policy options are assessed in a transparent way, third, the chosen strategy is implemented and evaluated, and finally, the findings are fed back into the system to improve the policy in the future (Nutley and Webb 2000). In reality such instrumental use of evaluation findings is rare since the policy process is much more complex (Hunter 2003). A wide range of other factors, such as fiscal stringency, shifts in ideology and values, the failure of existing systems, and intellectual fashion, inform policy decisions (Davies and Howden-Chapman, 1996). Policy-making is perhaps better thought of as 'ethereal', 'diffuse, haphazard and somewhat volatile' (Lomas 2000, p. 140), and as a result, different kinds of evidence may be useful at different points in time (Black 2001). Moreover, policy-makers consider a much wider range of evidence than scientific research and evaluation in their decision-making. For example the Cabinet Office's guide to professional policy-making defines evidence in a much broader way as shown in Box 2.2.

Box 2.2 Evidence in policy-making

Good quality policy making depends on high quality information derived from a variety of sources – expert knowledge; existing domestic and international research; existing statistics; stakeholder consultation; evaluations of previous polices, new research, if appropriate; or secondary sources, including the internet. Evidence can also include analysis of the outcomes from consultations, costings of policy options and the results from economic and statistical modelling.

There is a tendency to think of evidence as something that is only generated by major pieces of research. In any policy area there is a great deal of critical evidence held in the minds of both front-line staff ... and those to whom policy is directed.

Source: Strategic Policy Making Team (SPMT) (1999, paras 7.1 and 7.22) quoted in Nutley and Webb (2000)

Given these kinds of issues, Nutley and colleagues (2002) suggest that evidence-based policy is a 'glib' term that 'can obscure the sometimes limited role that evidence can, does or even should play' (pp. 1–2). Instead they argue that it would be better to think in terms of 'evidence-influenced' or 'evidence-aware' policy.

Weiss (1995a) argues that evaluations are used in the policy process, but in less direct ways: to mobilise support and legitimise decisions policy-makers have already made; to act as a warning when social problems are growing beyond acceptable limits; to provide theory and evidence about action that could be taken and to provide enlightenment by contributing general ideas and concepts to improve understanding of the policy terrain.

Conducting evaluations within an evidence-based framework has implications for the nature of the study. In many of the recent large pilot evaluations established by central government, the research question has not been *does the initiative work*, but *what aspects of it work, why and for whom?* In addition, evaluators have been expected to undertake development, learning and sometimes management roles in relation to the pilots, as well as more traditional evaluation tasks (Martin and Sanderson 1999; Evans et al. 2001). The emphasis in this approach to evaluation is on developing the interventions, demonstrating the benefits that flow from them and disseminating models of good practice (Martin and Sanderson 1999). A spectrum of involvement by evaluators in these kinds of processes can be seen to have developed. While there was little evidence of this in the national evaluation of total purchasing pilots (commissioned in the final years of the Conservative government) (Evans et al. 2001), there was much more explicit demand for this kind of approach within the national evaluation of the New Deal for Communities (NDC Evaluation Team 2002), while the design of the national evaluation of the Children's Fund is explicitly aimed at offering developmental support to case study partnerships (http://www.ne-cf.org.uk, accessed 21 January 2005). Some commentators have questioned whether it is possible to bring these different roles – of impact assessment and iterative policy learning – together in the same pilot projects and evaluations (Martin and Sanderson 1999).

A range of issues arise from this, which presented key challenges for the HAZ evaluation. First, the policies subject to evaluation were constantly evolving, both in response to changes in central government's aspirations and local experience on the ground (Barnes, J. et al. 2003). Moreover, decisions about the fate of pilots are often taken before evaluation findings are produced in response to a wide range of other factors (Martin and Sanderson 1999; Evans et al. 2001). While evaluators often try to inform these debates with interim reports and ongoing dialogue and feedback, there is a tension between producing information when policy-makers want it and producing findings when the data have been collected and appropriately analysed (Evans et al. 2001). Researchers have sought to deal with these tensions in a number of ways. For example, in an evaluation of Scottish health demonstration projects, there was an explicit transition period built into the plans to allow for evaluation findings to be produced, and learning from them to feed into the second phase of development (McVea 2003). More generally, this emphasis on iterative policy learning requires a much more interactive relationship between policy-makers and researchers, both nationally and locally. This needs to be an informed two-way process so that it does not lead to pressure on evaluators to identify 'lessons learnt' for future policy scenarios that can take them outside of the limits of their evaluation findings (Geva-May and Pal 1999). Both advocates (Macintyre et al. 2001) and critics (Klein 2000) of evidence-based policy warn evaluators and commentators of the dangers of doing this.

Secondly, the social programmes initiated by the New Labour government had long-term objectives, but the pilots and their evaluations often covered much shorter periods. Given these constraints, evaluations often focus on implementation and process issues rather than final outcomes (Sanderson 2000). There is considerable value in this (Mackenbach 2003). Much can be learnt for future policy initiatives by developing a better understanding of how policies are implemented in practice, how they generate effects and how these depend on the contextual circumstances and the interrelationships with other polices and processes (Sanderson, 2000). Nevertheless, there is often still an unrealistic expectation within the relevant policy communities that such evaluations will be able to make substantive statements about the impact of the initiative on final outcomes.

Third, the complexity of many of these programmes means that a wide range of stakeholders are involved. In assessing the 'impact' of an initiative, across a whole host of possible process and outcome measures, it is important to consider that different stakeholders – policy-makers, managers, front-line staff and users – both nationally and locally, will have different values about different kinds of achievements (Sullivan et al. 2004). It is often difficult for evaluators to accurately reflect these competing views and values in their analyses (Martin and Sanderson 1999). The complex and dynamic nature of these initiatives also means that it is not possible to define precisely what the initiative consists of, that 'what it is' changes over time, and means different things to different people (Barnes, M. et al. 2003b).

Finally, the emphasis on providing development support for the pilot sites is a new role for evaluators, which they are not necessarily skilled to do, and that may compromise their independence. Again, a spectrum of approaches can be seen within current evaluations. For example, while there was modest development support for the initiative itself sought from the national HAZ evaluation team (see Chapter 4), providing detailed technical support to the initiatives was a key feature of the evaluation brief for the NDC (NDC Evaluation Team 2002). There is a potential tension between having a more interactive and supportive role with the pilot sites and central government, and maintaining the separateness of the evaluation to ensure independent assessments can be made (Evans et al. 2001), especially when different stakeholders may place very different values on alternative outcomes from the initiative and the evaluation.

Given these kinds of issues, Klein (2000) questions whether investment in rigorous scientific evaluations will actually produce useful results within policy-makers' timeframes, and argues instead for simple reportage and analysis of existing data. However, Weiss (1998a) does not take such a pessimistic view and argues that evaluation can and should still make a valuable contribution to policy-making, but to do so evaluators need to plan their study clearly in terms of what they want it to be used for, by whom and in what circumstances. The evaluation approach adopted in relation to HAZ is discussed in Chapter 4.

Conclusion

The HAZ initiative was one of the first of a raft of policies that reflected New Labour's aspirations to transform the public sector and achieve more socially just outcomes for citizens. This involved recognising the interconnectedness of policy problems, not least that of poor health and health inequalities, and the consequent need for effective collaboration across agencies and sectors if they were to be successfully addressed. Government at all levels also needed to develop a new relationship with citizens who should be included as partners in delivering policy objectives, and action needed to be focused and targeted in those areas most adversely affected by previous policy failures. Policies should be subject to evaluation and review to ensure they were delivering what was intended.

As a very early initiative HAZ was described as a radical break with the past and those areas that were given HAZ status were seen as 'trailblazers', marking a path that others would follow. What was not anticipated was the speed with which the highway of mainstream service delivery would be expected to adopt many of the characteristics that distinguished HAZ and other special programmes, thus leaving the HAZ trail out in the cold. Chapter 3 describes how we aimed to evaluate the HAZ endeavour, and describes some of the challenges involved.

Evaluating policy and practice

Designing the national HAZ evaluation

Mhairi Mackenzie and Michaela Benzeval

Introduction

HAZs were one of a range of initiatives established by New Labour that encouraged local agencies to work in partnership and, through experimenting with new models of service delivery, to establish 'what works' (Martin and Sanderson 1999). They were initially launched as pilot projects (Dobson 1997) and as such HAZs were expected to contribute in a range of ways to the new emphasis on evidence-based policy-making. To support learning from HAZs, local partnerships were required to undertake their own evaluations of their activities and at the same time the DH commissioned a national evaluation.

In this chapter we explore some of the main evaluation frameworks available to those charged with assessing the value of policy programmes and describe the approach adopted by the national HAZ evaluation team.

Approaches to evaluation

If the salience of evaluation within current thinking about policy-making at least at a rhetorical level is accepted, then it is important to consider whether the approaches and tools that evaluators bring to learning are fit for purpose. This section briefly rehearses the limitations inherent within traditional evaluation paradigms before discussing the promise offered by the new generation of theory and realist based approaches to policy learning.

Using experimentation: the positivist paradigm

Rossi and Wright (1987) identify the 1960s and early 1970s as the 'Golden Age' of evaluation in the United States. During this period federal and state governments made significant investments in a range of policies and programmes to reduce inequalities with a particular focus on education, training and employment (Maynard 2000). For the academic psychologists and economists who took on the mantle of evaluator, the paradigm of preference, in parallel with that operating within the medical field, was the randomised controlled trial (RCT).

The aim of such evaluation was to measure the net impact of a given programme by controlling for contextual variables so that policy decisions might be taken about whether or not to continue the programme. The evaluator was a technical expert with skills in manipulating variables and measuring effects in an objective way. This positivist paradigm was hoped to provide a means of obtaining value neutral assessments of whether a programme had achieved its goals and of whether a policy was effective. As Rossi and Wright (1987, p. 51) observe, 'to many social scientists of a technocratic bent, the randomised field experiment promised to replace our bumbling trial and error approaches to forging social policy with a more self-consciously rational "experimenting society".'

The reality, however, was that for ethical, legal and technical reasons randomisation outside the clinical field proved difficult, if not impossible. The solution for researchers working within this paradigm was to rely on the quasi-experimental approach, devised by Campbell and Stanley (1966), as a means of testing the success of a range of health subsidy, educational improvement and job training programmes (Maynard 2000).

These experimental approaches are not, however, believed to have made good their early promise and their critics raise a wide array of objections.

First, the policy lessons generated by the approaches were felt to be disappointing because the findings in relation to the net impact of the various programmes were either negative or inconclusive. Rossi and Wright (1987), note that 'the key lesson from the Golden Age is that the expected effects of social programs hover near zero, a devastating discovery for the social reformers of the time' (p. 48). Sorensen and colleagues (1998), for example, describe the contradictory and negligible impacts made by community health heart interventions. For Pawson and Tilley (1997), working in the United Kingdom, there is a parallel mismatch between the promise and the reality of what the experimental approach can deliver; thus 'the underlying logic ... seems meticulous, clear-headed and militarily precise, and yet findings seem to emerge in a typically non-cumulative, low-impact, prone-to-equivocation sort of way' (p. 8).

Secondly, critics point to inherent inadequacies of experimental methodologies in addressing the types of complex questions that policy makers need answered. In other words, whilst an experimental approach can give an answer to the question of whether there is a statistically significant difference in a selected set of outcomes between an experimental and control area, it cannot indicate why this has happened. Where no differences are found, or where different evaluations of similar programmes throw up conflicting evidence, there is an absence of richer learning about why this is the case. The bluntness of the evaluation tool prevents sharp distinctions being made about who an initiative works for, how it works, and, under

what circumstances – in short, the contents of the black box and its recipients remain a mystery. In addition, the black box is viewed not only as
whole and indivisible but also as an entity separate from its own social and
political context. Context, within this paradigm, offers a raft of variables
that must be controlled for rather than the arena within which a policy
intervention takes life and provides meaning to its recipients.

Another criticism of experimental approaches is their attempt to strip evaluation of values (Scriven 1984; Guba and Lincoln 1988; House and Howe
1999). Evaluations are viewed as technical affairs rather than judgements
located, at least partly, within a cultural context. Central to this last criticism
is the view that knowledge derived from evaluation is itself contested. It is
from this stance that more constructionist approaches to evaluation derive.

Using qualitative approaches: where realism meets social constructionism

For those whose evaluation practice is driven predominantly by an adherence
to qualitative modes of inquiry, there is a distinction to be made between what
Guba and Lincoln (1988) refer to as third and fourth generation approaches
to evaluation. This distinction rests on whether or not the evaluator is
believed to offer an objective assessment of the value of a social programme.

Fourth generation or constructionist models, based on value-pluralism,
are fundamentally relativist and postmodern. In other words, they contest
the existence of an objective reality and believe that no set of values should
be privileged over another. This paradigm is concerned with reflecting back
conflicting realities to stakeholders in a non-judgemental way:

> equity demands that the constructions, claims, concerns, and issues that
> stem from each value pattern be solicited and honored ... the evaluator
> must project an ... insider's view for each audience, and be prepared to
> accept it at face value unless and until that audience itself determines to
> change it.
>
> (Guba and Lincoln 1988, p. 77)

However, amongst many who adopt both qualitative methods and a plural-
ist tendency within a realist paradigm (for example, Scriven 1984; House
and Howe 1999) there is a disquiet about the view that evaluators should
refrain from making value judgements. For Scriven there is, in addition, an
objection to the principle of multiple realities:

> although we may reject the existence of a single correct description, we
> should not abandon the idea that there is an objective reality, though it
> may be a very rich one that cannot be exhaustively described.
>
> (Scriven 1984, p. 59)

In opposition to experimentalists (who, as discussed earlier, view their purpose as the measurement of facts that are intrinsically value-free and therefore objective) and constructionists (who believe neither fact nor value to be testable and real), House and Howe (1999) advocate an alternative that they describe as deliberative and democratic. This approach is based on three main principles: inclusion, dialogue and deliberation. Essentially, within this model the evaluator has a *democratic* duty to seek the views and perspectives of key stakeholders and to redress imbalances in power in presenting findings.

As with the constructionist approaches these views need to be accessed through a process of critical dialogue. Where this approach departs from its more constructionist relatives is that the values within these views should be subjected to reasoned deliberation. House and Howe (1999) argue that this approach can then deliver an objectively verifiable evaluation but, interestingly, define objectivity in a way which would look to positivists a lot like subjectivity since valuing remains an integral part of the evaluator's role:

> The sense of objectivity we wish to reject explicitly is the positivist notion that objectivity depends on stripping away all conceptual and value aspects and getting down to the bedrock of pristine facts. Rather, being objective, in our sense means working toward unbiased statements through the procedures of the discipline, observing the canons of proper argument and methodology, maintaining a healthy scepticism, and being vigilant to eradicate sources of bias.
>
> (House and Howe 1999, p. 9)

Although there are important philosophical distinctions to be made between the deliberative democratic or realist approach and the broader constructionist school, the need for careful and critical methods for eliciting and representing competing perspectives remains central to all utilizing qualitative approaches.

From a policymaker's point of view, there are more practical criticisms to be made of the constructionist approach. If the RCT is altogether too blunt an instrument for understanding why social programmes do or do not work, then the constructionist instrument is arguably too carefully focused on the particular task alone and, as a result, is of little use for macro-level policy making. Pawson and Tilley (1997) caricature this as follows:

> Naturalists thus acknowledge the significance of the context on constraining the actions, standpoints and negotiations of stakeholders. They regard these circumstantial features as being likely to vary between the past, present, and future as well as the here, there, and everywhere

and they seek to resolve the dilemma by trying to cope only with the here and now.

(Pawson and Tilley 1997, p. 22)

Both of the broad paradigms discussed so far take a particular epistemological stance on the types of data to be collected, the methods that should be utilized, and, how evaluation findings should impact on their audience. They might be characterized as being either methods or data driven approaches to evaluation. In contemporary policy evaluations (for example the National Evaluation of Sure Start – NESS, 2000) they commonly live under the same roof, despite their different underlying assumptions about the nature of knowledge. By doing so, they attempt to bring both scientific rigour and data richness to bear on a particular series of evaluation questions.

A third broad group of evaluation approaches takes its impetus not from a particular methodological preference or from a desire to collect certain types of data but from the underlying theory of the evaluation as understood by its key stakeholders.

Theory-based approaches to evaluation

Macintyre and colleagues (2001), in a review of the types of evidence used to influence policy on tackling health inequalities within the United Kingdom, lament the lack of rigorous systematic reviews informing the design of complex interventions. The complex nature of social programmes, however, means that generating useful policy learning is fraught with difficulty. Connell and Kubisch (1998) in their discussion of what they term comprehensive community-based initiatives (CCIs) highlight a number of features of such programmes that make them especially resistant to evaluation using traditional approaches.

First, such initiatives can be characterized as being both horizontally and vertically complex. Horizontal complexity refers to the current imperative for initiatives to work jointly through partner organizations that have potentially different responsibilities and goals. This complexity is exacerbated when the intervention is expected to impact at the level of individuals, communities and organizations (vertical complexity). As Davey Smith and colleagues (2001) point out, 'the sort of evidence gathered on the benefits of interventions aimed at individuals may not help in guiding policies directed towards reducing health inequalities' (Davey Smith et al. 2001, p. 184).

Secondly, such initiatives commonly have the goal of building community capacity, both as an end in its own right and as a means of affecting change. This is notoriously difficult to achieve both in terms of practice and in terms of measurement.

Thirdly, rather than viewing success as being independent of political, economic and cultural context, these initiatives are explicitly expected to incorporate these contextual features within their programme planning. Clearly this has implications for experimental approaches that rely heavily on the principle of controlling for potentially confounding variables. The problem of experimental control is compounded by the fact that initiatives, which cover communities, are expected to reach population saturation so that the potential for identifying suitable controls within the intervention area is diminished.

Connell and Kubisch (1998) also note that CCIs are designed to be flexible over time and are therefore dynamic entities rather than temporally and geographically consistent interventions. In addition, the national policy environments within which they are located are often fluid and movable feasts. Not only does policy change in relation to the intervention areas themselves but also early lessons from initiatives are used to push forward policy in other geographical areas. In order to do such interventions justice, therefore, evaluations need to invest effort in capturing and understanding the changing context within which they are located. Given all of this, the potential for policy contamination of possible control areas is considerable.

An additional problem is that complex initiatives are set up to deal with the biggest and most intractable social and economic problems of contemporary society. If they are to be successful then their long-term outcomes can unfold only beyond the lifespan of both the initiative and its evaluation. Not only is the cost of high-quality outcome data prohibitively expensive for state-funded evaluation (Martin and Sanderson 1999), but also Lindholm and Rosen (2000) have argued that an increasing number of confounding variables intervene over time between a community-based programme and its long-term outcomes (such as mortality). Such outcomes are particularly prone to dilution bias for a number of reasons. First, population mobility out of and into the study area after an intervention may reduce its assessed impact as not all members of the community whose final outcomes are measured will have received the intervention. Secondly, in some cases, non-interventions risk factors may change over time affecting the outcome in either the intervention or control area. For example in the Multiple Risk Factor Intervention Trial (MRFIT) study, there was a much greater reduction in coronary heart disease (CHD) deaths in control areas than expected after 7.5 years as a result of falls in smoking and other risk factors, which reduced the apparent effect of the intervention (MRFIT Research Group 1982). As a result, Lindholm and Rosen (2000) argue that community interventions should be evaluated by measuring changes in intermediate risk factors close to the interventions that have been shown to be causal in other research.

We are inclined to concur with Schorr (1998) that whilst comprehensive initiatives may be the most promising interventions in terms of impact they are also the least likely to be understood using traditional evaluation methods. Indeed, even those researchers who espouse RCTs as the gold standard recognize that the evaluation of complex interventions require a period of theory generation before commencing to randomisation (Campbell et al. 2000). Campbell and colleagues propose a model of evaluation that starts from theory generation in order to clarify the purpose of the intervention before moving, in a linear or cyclical fashion, to modeling and experimental phases. Although designed as a means of improving learning from the implementation of complex interventions it fails to take into account, however, the fact that most policy interventions do not reach a point of stability but, react to and interact with, their local and national context.

Theory-based evaluation has evolved to address these challenges. An early approach under this banner is that of Wholey (1983), who believed that a major problem for evaluators was that initiatives were not established in such a way as to make them amenable to evaluation. The concept of evaluability assessment was therefore developed whereby, in advance of undertaking a formal evaluation, the evaluator examines the reasoning underlying the links between a programme's activities and its anticipated outcomes.

This early work has been expanded greatly by the work of the Aspen Institute's Roundtable on Comprehensive Community Initiatives (Connell et al. 1995; Fulbright-Anderson et al. 1998) and forms the basis of the Theories of Change (ToC) model of evaluation.

The approach is most simply defined as 'a systematic and cumulative study of the links between activities, outcomes and contexts of the initiative' (Connell and Kubisch 1998, p. 35), and is undertaken with the evaluator working with key stakeholders to elicit their theories of why, and under what set of contextual circumstances, a particular initiative is anticipated to lead to the desired long-term outcomes (the way in which a Theory of Change is elicited in practice is highlighted in Box 3.1). This approach encompasses two distinct types of theory – implementation theory that focuses on how an intervention is put into practice as advocated by Wholey (1983) and Chen (1990), and programme theory that explains the rationale underlying the intervention's design as advocated by Weiss (1995b).

It is important here to understand that theory is not used as a term for grand formal reasoning, rather it is the more nebulous form of thinking that people do as a matter of course in planning and implementing solutions to problems. Weiss (1995b) captures this as follows:

> Theories represent the stories that people tell about problems and how they can be solved. Laypeople as well as professionals have stories about the origins and remedies of social problems ... These stories, whether they arise from stereotypes, myths, journalism, or research knowledge, whether they are true or false, are potent forces in policy discussion ... to the extent that evaluation can directly demonstrate the hardiness of some stories (theories) and the frailty of others, it will address the underlying influences that powerfully shape policy discourse.
>
> (Weiss 1995b, p. 72)

Box 3.1 Undertaking a Theory of Change

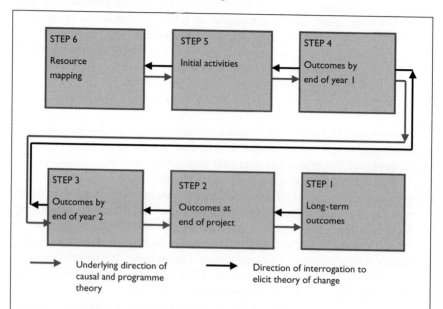

Source: adapted from Connell and Kubisch (1998)

To elicit the Theory of Change underlying a planned programme, the evaluator works with a wide range of stakeholders in a collaborative manner. Part of the evaluator's role is to facilitate the articulation of the relevant theories and to highlight conflicting and discrepant theories. To help capture expectations of change, stakeholders are asked to focus explicitly on the following steps and to reflect on the contextual factors that influence their decision-making.

- *Step 1:* The focus here is on the long-term vision of an initiative and is likely to relate to a timescale that lies beyond the timeframe of the initiative. For example, a HAZ might have a long-term vision of eradicating inequalities in premature mortality from CHD. This aim should be closely linked to evidence of a local or national problem.
- *Step 2:* Having agreed the ultimate aim of the programme, stakeholders are encouraged to consider the *necessary* outcomes that will be required by the end of the programme if such an aim is to be met in the longer term. Within HAZ these programme outcomes might involve setting a target in relation to reducing premature mortality.

(continued)

- *Steps 3 and 4:* Stakeholders are then asked to articulate the types of outputs and short-term outcomes that will help them to achieve the specified targets. These might include the establishment of user consultation groups, joint partnership planning structures, reductions in differential access to services and reductions in smoking.
- *Step 5:* At this stage those involved with the programme consider the most appropriate activities or interventions required to bring about the required change. The establishment of smoking cessation clinics or the development of accessible rehabilitation services might be proposed.
- *Step 6:* Finally, stakeholders are required to consider the resources that can realistically be brought to bear on the planned interventions. These will include staff and organisational capacity, the existence of supportive networks and facilities as well as financial capability.

Following a collective and iterative process the resulting ToC, if it is to be a useful, must fulfil a set of pre-specified criteria: these are that it must be plausible, doable, testable and meaningful. Firstly, then, the ToC that is elicited should be interrogated to ensure that the underlying causal theory is one that is acceptable to stakeholders either because of its existing evidence base or because it seems likely to be true in a normative sense. Secondly, the implementation theory itself should be questioned to ensure that timescales, financial resources and capacities add up to the aspirations of the programme. Thirdly, the ToC needs to be articulated in such a way that it can be open to evaluation; this is possible only where there is a high degree of specificity concerning the outcomes of the programme. Finally, the programme needs to be locally meaningful and of sufficient priority in relation to the investment that is planned; this latter issue is largely an economic question.

Connell and Kubisch (1998) see the attractions of theory-based approaches as being threefold. First, the approach, if undertaken during the design phase, can 'sharpen the planning and implementation of an initiative' (p. 17).

Secondly, the approach helps to facilitate the process of developing an evaluation framework by specifying the measurement and data collection components of the initiative. Thirdly, it is argued that where a Theory of Change has been articulated and collectively agreed during the early life of the initiative, then problems associated with causal attribution can be lessened.

The Theories of Change approach is only one of a number of frameworks to evaluation that stresses the need to open the black box of an intervention or programme and to understand it within context. Another theory-based approach that is gaining in popularity is *Realistic Evaluation* (Pawson and Tilley 1997). Its central tenet is that 'it is not programs as such that work but the generative mechanism that they release by way of providing reasons and resources to change behaviour' (p. 36). This is partly because social programmes are generally loose confederations of plans, policies and activities and therefore to consider them to be a united whole is facile. Secondly, they are implemented in a variety of pre-existing contexts and communities that represent a rich interweaving of potentially relevant factors such as social capital, race relations and organisational cohesiveness.

From a policy point of view, the evaluation findings that matter are those that provide judgements about what worked where, with whom and why. Thus, Pawson and Tilley (1997) argue that the key role of evaluation should be to better understand the relationships which exist between specific contexts, the intervention and its outcomes and, in particular, to understand the mechanisms by which an intervention leads to certain outcomes within certain contexts. Not only will the implementation of a social programme be implemented differently in different areas but also there will be conflicting theories about the mechanisms by which it will be thought to impact on key outcomes. Realistic evaluation, therefore, shares with Theories of Change a concern for both context and the testing of theory. The approaches are, however, far from synonymous in how they conceptualise theory and in the scale of the programmes within which they are believed to be best suited to generating learning. (A comparative critique of the two approaches is beyond the scope of this chapter; a summary of some of the key distinctions can be found in Pawson and Tilley (1997).)

Adopting a theory-based approach does not in itself preclude the use of particular quantitative or qualitative methods. Advocating the need to start from a position of understanding programme theory, the general approaches are a relatively broad church when it comes to selecting methods. Evaluators such as Owen and Rogers (1999) set out potentially useful ways of blending routine data, observational, documentary, interview, survey and outcome data. They show how the various stages of the evaluation process (from the programme design, through programme clarification and monitoring to impact assessment) ask different questions and therefore necessitate different types of data.

Whilst there remain important questions about the extent to which current social programmes do lend themselves to meaningful evaluation and the role that evaluators should play in increasing 'evaluability', it would at least seem plausible that a theory-based approach is a useful way to begin the process of determining the key questions that should be addressed. These questions then become the means of selecting appropriate research methods and tools. The chapter now turns to the way in which this was negotiated within the national evaluation of HAZ.

The national evaluation of HAZs

Early plans

In the spring of 1998 the Department of Health (DH) invited applications to undertake the central or national evaluation of HAZs. Its key require-ments were for the national evaluation to:

- address strategic issues of importance for central policy on Health Action Zones and for the wider policy agenda of *The New NHS* White Paper and the *Our Healthier Nation* Green Paper
- contribute valuable lessons to support HAZ development locally (although it made clear that this did not mean the development of specific individual HAZs) (DH R&D Division 1998).

The research brief highlighted the fact that HAZs were expected to have a life of five to seven years and that the central evaluation would need to be capable of assessing interim achievements as well as a longer term impact. Beyond this the DH recognized the very wide scope of what HAZs might try to do. Even so it was expected that the evaluation should be concerned with assessing processes as well as outcomes and impact, and to ascertain how, as well as whether, objectives are achieved.

Within the guidance the DH also set out a number of strategic themes that the evaluation should cover:

- improving health and reducing health inequalities
- restructuring and integrating services for improved health outcomes
- securing improved value for money from all available resources
- building and sustaining partnerships
- involving and empowering local communities to achieve sustainable development
- exploiting freedoms available to HAZs, forging innovation, bringing together policy and implementation and influencing central policy development.

Box 3.2 The model of HAZs

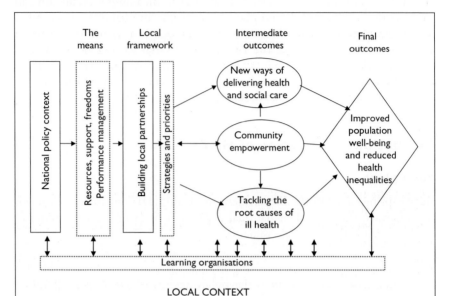

Figure 3.1 A model of Health Action Zones
Source: Judge et al. (1999)

As Figure 3.1 illustrates, within the national policy context, some particular policy levers were developed for HAZs. These were the means by which HAZs operated and included both opportunities, in terms of the resources, freedoms and support, and obligations, most clearly articulated in a performance management framework. Within the bounds of these two policy envelopes, each HAZ created its own local framework. This had two key foundations: the partnership relationships and the strategy and priorities that were developed to achieve their goals. The way in which partnerships were formed and worked together to assess their needs, develop their strategies and delivery their services was fundamental to the success of the HAZ initiative. Crucially, they had to decide on an appropriate balance between the different intermediate outcomes: new ways of delivering health and social care; community empowerment; and, tackling the root causes of ill health. These outcomes were goals in their own right, but also represented the means of attaining the final outcomes, which were improved population health and well being, and a reduction in inequalities within them. Finally, the government emphasised that HAZs should be learning organisations.

(continued)

The initial bid for the evaluation was organised around the components of the model across a number of different universities and organisations, which drew together individuals and groups with the wide range of knowledge and experience necessary to cover all of these issues. Although the requirements of the national evaluation were changed during the commissioning process and in response to the changing policy context of HAZs, these key components remained important building blocks of the national evaluation throughout.

We used these themes, together with other relevant policy statements and information from the bids for HAZ status, to develop a model to guide the evaluation, which is shown in Box 3.2. This model was considered crucial to managing the evaluation of the HAZ initiative, which covered such wide-ranging activities and processes, in order to provide flexibility over time but within a coherent and conceptually led approach.

In addition, in the bid for the national evaluation we outlined a number of important elements that have guided the approach of the evaluation over time. First, we argued that a 'Theories of Change' approach to the evaluation was the most appropriate way to develop meaningful policy lessons from the HAZ experience. Drawing on the general literature, as described earlier in this chapter, it was decided that the national evaluation should identify what features of HAZ status and investments worked in what circumstances.

Secondly, given the complexity of the challenges in the communities in which HAZs were established and the considerable policy contamination that was occurring with other areas, it was decided that the identification of controls was inappropriate. Instead, we planned to undertake comparisons within the HAZ endeavour, examining changes in HAZs over time and investigating different approaches adopted to particular problems in different contexts and assessing their success. In addition, we aimed to set the HAZ experience within a broader comparative context through a range of other policy evaluations that were being undertaken by the proposed team simultaneously.

Thirdly, we felt that it was important to combine monitoring with focused evaluations to provide an overall assessment of the HAZ programme. To do this we planned to examine specific important features or mechanisms in different contexts across the HAZs rather than evaluate individual HAZs in detail.

Fourthly, one important issue discussed in depth in the bid was how to study the impact of the HAZ initiative given that it was unlikely that changes in final health outcomes would occur during the lifetime of the evaluation. Building on theory of change ideas and the need to identify intermediate outcomes important to the HAZ endeavour, we felt that three questions were important:

- What changes could be identified in the way in which services were delivered?
- What was the impact on people and places of reshaping services and interventions?
- How sustainable are policies and practices that were judged to be effective?

The different ways in which these questions were explored within the evaluation are discussed in more detail below.

The final principle that underpinned the approach of the national evaluation was that the evaluation itself should be a partnership with local evaluators and policy makers. We were strongly committed to supporting local evaluators. We held methodological workshops and tried to encourage and facilitate the use of common instruments and data collection. In addition, we felt that a central part of the evaluation was to provide constant feedback of the findings from the evaluation to assist the further development of the HAZ, and planned a range of mechanisms for this purpose.

Given the uncertainty surrounding the HAZ initiative and the type of national evaluation that was required by the DH, the commissioning process for the evaluation was considerably protracted, and in the final event the evaluation was commissioned in a number of phases. The delays and uncertainty in the commissioning process, together with other aspects of the design requirements and general expectations, created a range of problems for the national evaluation. The implications of these problems for commissioning national evaluations in the future are discussed in Chapter 9. Nevertheless, the principles described above continued to guide the overall approach of the evaluation as it developed over time.

The general approach

The national evaluation of Health Action Zones formally began in January 1999. The first priority was to conduct a scoping exercise and to make recommendations about the future direction of research (Judge et al. 1999). Following detailed negotiations with the DH a formal contract for the next phase of the evaluation was agreed for three years from 2000, with the research beginning in the summer of that year. The overarching aim of the national evaluation was to identify and assess the conditions in which strategies to build capacity for local collaboration resulted in the adoption of change mechanisms that led to the modernisation of services and a reduction in health inequalities. It was recognized that detailed research on the management of change might be possible only in a sample of HAZs. Nevertheless, there was a general requirement to maintain contact with all twenty-six HAZs, to establish effective links with regional performance management arrangements, to synthesise and to coordinate the work of local evaluators, and to invest in dissemination efforts of various kinds.

The evaluation was divided into four broad modules, which were undertaken by different research groups within the evaluation team:

- monitoring all twenty-six HAZs and providing development support (Social Policy, Glasgow)
- building capacity for collaboration (Birmingham) – working with five case study HAZs
- whole systems change (Public Health, Glasgow and Queen Mary, London) – working with eight case study HAZs
- tackling inequalities in health (Queen Mary, London) – working with three case study HAZs.

Within each of the case study modules, efforts were made to identify stakeholders' theories of change at a number of different levels:

- *strategic:* for example, overall theories about how to tackle health inequalities, improve child health or develop partnership working
- *meso:* for example, workstreams focusing on addressing local employment problems or promoting community involvement
- *project level:* for example, community cafes for people with mental health problems, culturally sensitive exercise programmes, or initiatives to promote secondary prevention of heart disease in disadvantaged areas.

The aim was to develop a better understanding of the various approaches adopted by different HAZs to achieve their goals, monitor their progress and identify the inhibiting and facilitating factors that were encountered in different local contexts in this endeavour.

The approach of each module is described in more detail in key evaluation reports (Bauld et al. 2001a; Barnes, M. et al. 2003b; Benzeval 2003a; Mackenzie et al. 2003). Although the evaluation team met periodically to discuss progress, in reality the separate modules were conducted independently, and the general approach, therefore, evolved in different ways within each of them. In part these differences reflected the disciplinary background and experiences of team members and in part the particular issues under investigation and how they developed within the particular HAZs collaborating with each module. For example, the modules attempted to work collaboratively with local evaluators to differing degrees. A central feature of the initial design of the building capacity for collaboration module was based on a co-research model. In the whole systems change module, exploring local strategies for evaluation and learning was a key part of the research focus, and there was close collaboration with local evaluators. However, in the tackling inequalities module, local evaluators were interviewed only to understand how they had examined issues around health inequalities, although other efforts were made to liaise with them to avoid duplication and share early findings.

More broadly, members of the national evaluation team worked with local evaluators to encourage them to use a Theories of Change approach. Not only was this believed to be the most appropriate approach in the complex circumstances that HAZs were operating within, but also it was hoped that it would be possible to identify generalisable policy lessons from across local evaluations. Local evaluators were not obliged to follow this approach, however, and a wide range of different local evaluations were conducted (Mackenzie et al. 2002).

The realities of using Theories of Change within the national HAZ evaluation

It was recognized from the outset that evaluations of initiatives such as HAZs are particularly problematic because of the complexities of the contexts in which they operate, the interventions and process that they introduce and the nature of the outcomes they wish to change. In addition, HAZs operated in a period of rapid and extensive policy change, which meant not only that HAZs were constantly evolving but also that the nature of the concerns of the evaluation's broader policy clients also changed over time. As Mays and colleagues note in their summary of the evaluation of total purchasing pilots, 'it seems almost inevitable that research-based evaluation of innovations can scarcely ever keep pace with changes in public policy' (Mays et al. 2001, p. 16).

As a result, the national HAZ evaluation team had to continuously make judgements about the balance between being true to the original research questions based on the starting point for HAZs, and adapting to the ever-changing circumstances of HAZs and the demands placed on them and the evaluation. To illustrate this, in this section we explore some of the key challenges that the evaluation faced, both practical and conceptual; how these affected its ability to employ a Theories of Change approach, the problems they created more generally; and, how the evaluation was adapted in response to them.

Problems in practice

The HAZ evaluation, like many others, encountered a range of practical problems that affected its progress in ways that had implications for the nature of the questions it could answer. These included the timing of the evaluation in relation to that of the initiative; the resources available to the evaluation given the scale and the geographic dispersal of the HAZs; and the expectations of the evaluation in comparison to what could realistically be achieved.

Like many evaluations, that of HAZ was commissioned only after the initiative itself had been established. Moreover, given the decision to undertaken a scoping exercise at the start the evaluation, the detailed work examining HAZs' change strategies did not begin until summer 2000, two years after the first wave HAZs had begun, and long after the implementation plans had been written. As a result, it was very difficult to elicit from stakeholders the theories that they had been operating with when they developed their strategies. In addition, it was about this time that morale within HAZs was particularly low as a result of the changes in priorities and funding announced by the government, described in Chapter 4. As a result, it sometimes proved difficult for the evaluation to engage with the wide range of stakeholders initially involved in the HAZs, as many had reduced the priority they attached to contributing to the HAZ endeavour by this point. This represents a general problem for policy evaluators and highlights the importance of capturing stakeholder theories at a point where there is both commitment to the general thrust of the programme and a willingness to sharpen their planning around it.

The resources available for the national evaluation were significant by traditional British evaluation standards but rather limited in comparison to many of the US evaluations from which the Theories of Change approach had emerged and in relation to contemporaneous UK policy evaluations such as that of Sure Start. An initial crude count of HAZ programmes and interventions identified more than 2000 separate projects (Judge et al. 1999). Clearly, it was impractical to examine even a selection of these with the level of detail needed to evaluate individual projects *per se*. Instead therefore, the national evaluation tried to examine HAZ objectives more strategically. However, even adopting this approach, it was not feasible for the detailed and interactive work that is required with stakeholders, to elicit their theories and to map appropriate milestones, to be undertaken. In addition, at this level identifying theories was even more difficult as stakeholders often had general, and perhaps contradictory, ideas about the directions of travel they wished to take, rather than specific causal or implementation pathways that they were trying to follow.

A further, and linked, complication was the geographic spread of the HAZs around England. Eliciting Theories of Change is an iterative process. Often the initial theories identified are fed back to stakeholders a number of times for refinement. This is often facilitated by close relationships being developed between stakeholders and the evaluators. However, given the distance between HAZs and the university bases of the evaluation teams, this close interactive relationship was not possible, making a Theories of Change approach that is grounded in the experiences of local stakeholders problematic. Certainly, experience in more local evaluations, where the initiative is smaller, has a clearer focus and allows a more interactive relationship between the evaluator and the local stakeholders, suggest that more progress can be made with this approach (Blamey et al., 2002) than was possible with the national evaluation of HAZs. In future, much more careful thought needs to be given to how national evaluations can undertake theory-based approaches that are grounded in the understanding of local players, by ensuring, for example, much closer relations between national and local evaluators or by having geographic satellites of national teams located near to local initiatives.

One final challenge that the evaluation experienced was that of meeting expectations. Initially, the HAZ initiative resulted in huge enthusiasm at the national and the local level, and as a result, there were high expectations about what it would achieve and hence what could be learnt from the evaluation. As a result, central policy makers and the HAZ community more generally had very varied, but considerable, expectations of what the HAZ evaluation could deliver and how quickly. For example, at one end of the spectrum of criticisms, there was an expectation among some parts of the HAZ community that the main focus of the national evaluation should be a before and after assessment of changes in final outcomes, at the other end, were frequent demands from central policy clients for instant lessons from the HAZ experience in terms of their relevance for a range of new policy initiatives. These expectations were often impossible, and/or inappropriate, for the national evaluation to try to meet. Nevertheless, this led to frustration and criticism of the national evaluation that was at times difficult to address. Managing expectations of what is and is not appropriate to expect from a national evaluation is clearly something that needs more explicit consideration and is arguably made more difficult where the lines between evaluation and programme mentor become blurred.

While these practical problems did present challenges for the evaluation in general, and for the adoption of a Theories of Change approach in particular, there were more fundamental issues associated with the HAZ initiative, which challenged the evaluation approach and led to a number of changes in how it was conducted.

Conceptual difficulties in utilizing Theories of Change within the national HAZ evaluation

In addition to the practical limitations that we have discussed, there are a number of features within the Theories of Change approach that make it conceptually problematic to apply.

These types of conceptual difficulty are starting to be discussed within a UK context (Sullivan et al. 2002; Barnes, M. et al. 2003a; Shaw and Crompton 2003; Mackenzie and Blamey 2005). For the purposes of this chapter, they are grouped into three interrelated issues: complexity; measuring impact; and the role of the evaluator and of evaluation more generally. These issues are discussed in turn in relation to the challenges that they raised for the National HAZ evaluation, the types of solutions that were developed, and the degree to which these were found to be effective.

Embracing complexity

We have already raised the question of complexity as a practical issue for evaluators. There is a wider question, however, about the extent to which Theories of Change can deal with the wide range of complexities that imbue health and social policy programmes. Complexity is a feature not only of the types of organizational structures that develop within particular locales but also of the way in which problems manifest themselves and of how their solutions are conceptualised and of the national and local processes of policy making (Chapman 2002). Breaking the so-called 'wicked problems' into their constituent parts runs the risk of losing some of the inherent complexity within systems of change.

The national evaluation attempted to capture complexity in a variety of ways:

- Within the evaluation as a whole there was a strong focus on context. From a practical and theoretical point of view this meant that the evaluation was shaped by an understanding that the local manifestation of a national initiative is largely determined by what has gone before and by the explicit decisions made to invest in building on, or reacting against, this context. All parts of the national evaluation viewed context to be important not only at the beginning of the initiative but throughout its lifespan and beyond. This approach recognized the fact that the relationship between the context and policy is two-way (Dahler-Larsen 2001) that is to say, HAZs affected, and were affected by, their local context in ways that hindered or facilitated the implementation of their activities over time.
- The evaluation was, in addition, focused primarily on the *process* of bringing about change. Thus, the need to build capacity for collaborative purposes, to engender whole systems change, and to purposefully develop strategies to tackle inequalities were recognized as central to the HAZ enterprise. Such processes could not be assumed to occur automatically as a result of implementation but needed to be evaluated in their own right.

- A conception of HAZs that was informed by the literature on whole systems and organizational development encouraged the evaluation to consider the views and theories of stakeholders and interventions at different levels within the planning and delivery of HAZ programmes of work. The evaluation, therefore, attempted to elicit Theories of Change at a range of different levels. The researchers that focused on capacity for collaboration, for example, elicited Theories of Change at macro, meso and micro levels within individual case study HAZs, whilst those investigating whole systems change and health inequalities sought views from stakeholders at strategic and operational levels of service planning.

- A further approach that was taken to understanding HAZs was to map the vast range of activities that the initiative was encompassing (undertaken during the scoping exercise and through the monitoring focus) and then to use this as a means of selecting topics as a means of studying change processes. Similarly, key findings from the substantive evaluation were used to shape the data collection instruments for regular monitoring across all twenty-six HAZs.

- The initial framework for the evaluation conceptualised building capacity for collaboration and bringing about whole systems change as stepping-stones en route to tackling health inequalities (See Figure 3.1 in Box 3.2). As the evaluation developed there was a move away from this relatively linear model to one where the various modules came to be viewed as a series of overlapping, but differently focused, lenses on the world of HAZ. In part this development arose from an increasing awareness that it is not possible to disentangle the nature of collaborative capacity from the ability to bring about whole systems change, nor to understand strategies for tackling inequalities in a contextual vacuum. The change in emphasis for the national evaluation made little practical difference but highlights the fact that complexity gives rise to potentially contested views of programme success (Barnes, M. et al. 2003a).

- Given this, the final outputs of the national evaluation represent a range of HAZ stories, at different levels, focused on different topics, from both an in depth and a comprehensive perspective, providing evaluative comments on past aspects of HAZ and broader government policy, and highlighting implications from HAZs' experiences for future policy at the local and the national levels.

Together, these approaches allowed the evaluation to view complexity as central to an understanding of the HAZ enterprise, however, a number of questions remain. Could this multilayered understanding of complexity have been reached without the Theories of Change framework and, indeed, is the Theories of Change model too linear to capture the subtleties of complex systems? We return to these issues in Chapter 9.

Measuring impact

Chapter 8 looks at the processes undertaken to measure the impact of the HAZ initiative and to provide an assessment of the type of impact made. Here we look briefly at some of the conceptual difficulties raised by the Theories of Change approach in relation to measuring impact and summarizes some of the approaches taken by the national evaluation team to augment the approach.

The Theories of Change approach suggests that, where theories are prospectively articulated and well specified, and where a programme's outcomes happen as predicted, then stakeholders, in the absence of competing explanations, will be happy to accept the causal nature of the initiative as it generates a level of evidence that is convincing to them (Connell and Kubisch 1998). This makes the task of the evaluator a more straightforward one but rests on the premise of there being a moderately good evidence base, effective planning and the availability of useful outcome data. In the context of the most complex initiatives this claim starts to look shaky for a number of reasons. First, as discussed in Chapter 6 and elsewhere (Judge and Mackenzie 2002; Mackenzie and Blamey 2005), HAZ stakeholders share with other similar initiatives an inability to articulate plans with the kind of level of detail that would be required to test the Aspen Institute's assertion. Secondly, this problem is not merely a practical one to be solved through greater technical support and a firmer grasp of the current evidence base on the effectiveness of specific interventions (although these would be helpful); rather, the complexity of the problems to be solved and the lack of rigorous evidence means that it is almost impossible for stakeholders to make precise predictions of impact in advance. This places interventions that are complex and poorly understood in a double bind: they have a poor existing evidence base; and, this in turn makes it more difficult for them to generate one for the future.

Measuring impact within individual HAZs was made more complex for the national evaluation because of the absence of primary data collection and the lack of timely secondary data. The types of efforts made by the team to address these gaps included the following.

- Performance measures, collected by individual case study HAZs as part of their reporting framework to the Department of Health, were reviewed. This strategy was impeded by a lack of consistency and of good quality data.

- Similarly, a brief analysis of changes over time in key indicators within the Public Health Common dataset was undertaken for HAZ and non-HAZ areas. This is described in Chapter 8. However, the most recently published data are for 2001, which allowed very little time for HAZs to have an impact on such outcomes.
- Within the evaluation, local perceptions of the success and impact of the HAZ within the key themes of the evaluation were considered. These are described in Chapters 5, 6 and 7. Here it was important to take account of the varying values that different stakeholders placed on the range of impacts identified. In relation to this, the evaluators augmented their assessment of HAZ progress through the utilisation of data collected through internal evaluation processes. The quality of such data was variable.
- In order to ensure that assessments of HAZ success were not constrained by a focus on the delivery of early plans or the national evaluation's main themes, all project managers were encouraged to retrospectively identify where their key areas of success had been. These examples of good practice were followed up in those HAZs that had not been utilised as case studies, by gathering the views of stakeholders and attempting to substantiate these through existing data sources (for example, routinely collected local data or reports produced by specially commissioned pieces of local evaluation). This analysis is described in Chapter 8. Once again, such data were variable.

Measuring impact will always be a difficult and contested business for evaluators and the national evaluation took a relatively eclectic approach to this task. A Theories of Change approach helped to maintain a focus for the evaluators on the explicit and implicit links between what HAZs aimed to do and what they achieved; whether it made a difference to the quality of the data that were available for scrutiny is a moot point.

The role of evaluation and of the evaluator

The final set of conceptual issues in the application of the Theories of Change approach relates to the assumptions that it makes about the role of both the evaluator and the evaluation more generally. At its heart it views evaluation as an empowering and democratic process, and sees the evaluator as a supportive and facilitative critic of an intervention. Within this it makes assumptions about the need for an *inclusive* process of theory articulation and the reaching of *consensus* on conflicting theories. Practical issues once again made it difficult to remain true to the approach within the national evaluation of HAZ. However, across the evaluation efforts were made to include a relatively broad range of stakeholders although, inevitably, these were chosen to represent existing constituents of the programmes. The modules also used differing levels of a co-research approach where decisions about how to include and what to focus on were made jointly with local evaluators and project managers. (This approach was most firmly embedded within the part of the evaluation focusing on building capacity for collaboration).

Nonetheless the Theories of Change approach to inclusion and consensus is not unproblematic even within a highly resourced evaluation scenario. Firstly, the approach does not explicitly deal with differential power relations that exist within the types of structures that have strategic responsibility for policy programmes, nor does it specify the criteria for determining who the legitimate stakeholders are and how one should deal with fundamentally conflicting theories (Sullivan et al. 2002). Secondly, some critics argue that evaluators using such an approach can be seduced into narrowing their evaluation focus to the limits of the intervention that is being introduced. In other words evaluators may focus on the effectiveness of implementing a particular programme on its self-specified goals rather than challenging the policy assumptions on which it is based (Sullivan et al. 2002; Shaw and Crompton 2003). Related to this criticism is the lack of clarity within the approach about whether the evaluator is limited to a technical expert who brings evaluation skills to the testing of programme theory or whether she brings substantive theory that is explicitly built into the development of an initiative's programme of activity. These questions are not raised *de novo* for evaluators by a Theories of Change approach but it perhaps made them more salient for those undertaking the national evaluation of HAZ.

Conclusion

The current climate for policy evaluation in the United Kingdom offers the promise of more fruitful relationships between those who make and implement policy, and those who seek to assess its impact and value. At the same time, that promise has proved illusory for a number of reasons that are practical, political and conceptual in nature. Theory-based approaches to evaluation offer one means of increasing the evaluability of social programmes and of augmenting the usefulness of evaluation findings for policymakers. In the case of the national evaluation of HAZ, the approach was loosely and variably used and met with challenges along the way that necessitated fairly extensive departures from the model as it was originally conceived.

Nonetheless, it helped to focus attention, across the evaluation, on the complexities of context as a defining feature of national policy initiatives and, as such generated learning about the implementation and evaluation of future policy programmes (Chapter 9). At a local level, the encouragement of the use of theory-based approaches helped to develop the capacity for evaluation, that arguably left a lasting legacy within the health community. Nationally, Theories of Change as an approach has become part of the establishment with, for example, the Office of the Deputy Prime Minister using it extensively in commissioning evaluation.

Chapter 4

The evolution of Health Action Zones

Linda Bauld, Jane Mackinnon and Julie Truman

Introduction

The Health Action Zone initiative began in 1998 and by 2003 most HAZs had ceased to exist. In their relatively short lifespan they were affected by a range of policy shifts driven by a complex series of events at local and national level. This chapter describes how HAZs evolved from promising beginnings to their submergence within wider public service reforms five years later. The chapter begins by examining the key characteristics of HAZs and the activities they chose to invest in. It then describes how relevant policy evolved during their lifetime and concludes with a discussion of the neighbourhood renewal and NHS reforms that eventually heralded the end of the initiative.

HAZ characteristics

The areas selected to become HAZs varied tremendously in relation to characteristics such as the nature of their population, their size and the type of inter-agency partnerships formed to lead them. However, all twenty-six zones shared a common history of deprivation and poor health. The majority were located in the more urban and industrial areas of England, which have some of the highest levels of deprivation in the country. Table 4.1 illustrates the level of deprivation in HAZs, using two different indices.

Table 4.1 Deprivation in Health Action Zones

| | Number of HAZ health authorities in each quartile | |
Deprivation quartiles	UPA Score 1991 Census	Index of Local Conditions 1991
Bottom 25% (least deprived)	0	0
25–50	7	5
50–75	12	13
Top 25% (most deprived)	15	16

Source: Public Health Common Dataset (1996); NIE (1998)

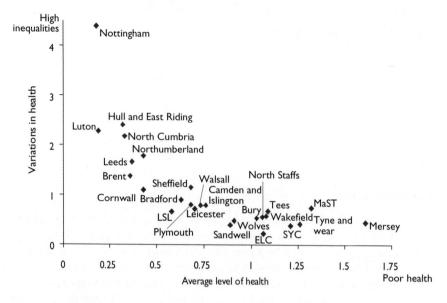

Figure 4.1 HAZ health and health inequalities: 2000 ward IMD health domain scores

Source: Benzeval (2003a, Figure 3)

As Table 4.1 illustrates, HAZ health authorities clearly dominated the more deprived quartiles of the distribution using two measures – Jarman's Underprivileged Area score and the 1991 Level of Local Conditions. HAZ health authorities accounted for fifteen out of the twenty-five most deprived health authorities on the UPA index and sixteen out of twenty-five using the Level of Local Conditions. In addition, HAZ authorities accounted for the top five most deprived health authorities on the UPA index and three of the top five authorities in the Level of Local Conditions Index.

This pattern of deprivation can also be seen using more recent data from the 2000 Index of Multiple Deprivation (IMD: DETR 2000b). The Index shows that a total of eighty-one of the hundred most deprived electoral wards in England were located within Health Action Zones. Half of all HAZ wards were in the most deprived quintile of wards in England, and less than 20 per cent of all HAZ wards were in the 50 per cent least deprived wards in the country (Adams et al. 2000).

It is also possible to illustrate the extent of the health inequalities problem that faced HAZs. Figure 4.1 shows the relationship between the average level of health and health inequalities between wards for each HAZ (based on the ward level health domain of the IMD: DETR 2000b).

The figure shows a negative association between the extent of inequalities between wards within a HAZ and its overall level of health (Benzeval

2003a). As the average level of ill health increases, the level of health inequalities falls, although this is clearly not a linear association. The HAZ with the highest level of health inequalities between its wards was Nottingham, while the smallest inequalities could be found in East London and the City HAZ. The best overall health among HAZs was in Luton, while the poorest health could be found in Merseyside. The four biggest HAZs, which were formed from multiple health authorities, also had the poorest levels of average health, and some of their constituent HAs had even more extreme levels.

Thus HAZs represented some of the most deprived areas of England with some of the poorest levels of ill health. Despite this common history, HAZs were complex entities that varied considerably in a number of other respects. Historical differences in their political structures and ways of working created different starting points for their work. In total, 13 million people in England lived in HAZ areas, representing over one-third of the population. Within HAZ areas, the population varied from 200,000 to 1.4 million. The geographical and organisational configuration of HAZs fell into five categories:

- multiple health authority, multiple local authority – such as Merseyside and Tyne and Wear
- single health authority, multiple local authority – including Nottingham, North Cumbria and others
- single health authority and multiple local authority – such as Camden and Islington and Teesside
- coterminous health and local authority – including Bradford, Sandwell, Wakefield and others
- sub health authority and local authority – such as Plymouth and Luton.

In addition to these organisational differences, HAZs demonstrated considerable variation in the size and scope of partnership structures they established. Some chose to have a dedicated steering group for the initiative (e.g. Merseyside), where others (e.g. Leeds) had a core team that was more integrated into existing structures of partner organisations through which representatives from the wider partnership group fed into the HAZ. Partners consisted of a wide variety of representatives from the statutory sector, voluntary and community groups, private sector and other public sector organisations such as the police. Further local variations amongst HAZs came in the form of demographic differences such as age structure, ethnic diversity and patterns of employment.

HAZ activities

In order to address the health needs of their varied populations, HAZs chose to invest in a wide range of projects and programmes. Information regarding these activities was provided in the HAZ implementation plans that were produced by each partnership at the start of the initiative. These plans were then modified following feedback from the Department of Health and later adapted locally as each zone developed.

A total of 214 'programmes' were identified across both first wave and second wave HAZs (Judge et al. 1999). Each programme described in the HAZ plans was allocated to one of seven major categories according to its main focus. These were:

- population groups
- health problems
- determinants of health
- health and social care
- community empowerment
- internal processes
- mixed.

Across both first wave and second wave HAZs, almost one-sixth of programmes (thirty-four) related primarily to improving the health of particular population groups. Of these almost half focused on young people, but a number of others targeted older people, black and ethnic minority groups and parents. A further twenty-eight programmes related to a specific health problem. The biggest group of programmes in this category focused on mental health as a priority. The remainder covered a range of issues such as accidents and violence, cardiovascular disease, diabetes, physical disabilities and others.

The largest proportion of initial programmes, almost one-third (sixty-one), was aimed at addressing the determinants of health. Across the HAZs the most common group of programmes in this category focuses on promoting healthy lifestyles, followed by improving employment, housing, education and tackling substance abuse. However, almost one-third of the root causes programmes were very general and attempt to tackle multiple causes in one programme.

The programmes that concentrated on health and social care accounted for just over one-tenth of initial HAZ activity. Many of these health and social care programmes had general aims, but others related particularly to improving primary care or community services, and a smaller number to hospital services and health promotion. Another one-tenth of programmes were centred on involving local communities. These included programmes that related to public involvement, community development, the provision of information to the public and other general community empowerment aims.

Not surprisingly at the outset of the initiative, there was a significant group of programmes that centred on the process of HAZ development.

Process programmes accounted for 13 per cent of all HAZ programmes and included strategy development, partnership development and evaluation and research. Finally, there were a small number of 'mixed' programmes that combined a range of approaches or which are focused on a particular area. Within these initial programmes, more than 2000 separate projects or activities were identified – 750 projects were specified by first wave HAZs in their plans, and 1036 by second wave HAZs (Judge et al., 1999).

The format of HAZ plans changed as the initiative developed. By 2000, the zones were expected to produce quarterly 'high-level statements' that described each programme and project and what progress they were making towards achieving their objectives. An analysis of this documentation in 2000 identified 264 separate high-level statements and within these 582 purposes, outlining the main focus of an activity undertaken by the HAZ (Bauld et al. 2001a). These purposes were categorised into the following key themes:

- population focus
- health problem/clinical focus
- process based
- goal based
- behaviour focus
- setting focus
- structural focus.

Box 4.1 provides an example of activities focused on one population group – children and young people.

Box 4.1 shows that HAZ projects related to children and young people took a variety of forms, from hospital-based interventions to community-based projects involving a wide range of partner organisations. This range of interventions was typical – projects focusing on another population group (such as older people) or health determinant (such as employment) demonstrated similar diversity. This wide variety of activity posed challenges for evaluation. It became almost impossible to easily describe in any simple manner what HAZs were doing at the level of the initiative as a whole, or indeed to adequately assess the extent of progress they were making in implementing their varied projects and programmes.

Evolving policy agenda

After the first wave of HAZs was launched in 1998, a number of important shifts in policy occurred that impacted on the initiative. These shifts went beyond the NHS to affect other organisations that formed a central part of HAZ partnerships, such as local government and voluntary organisations. The type of change experienced by HAZs was not unique – the zones

Box 4.1 Examples of activities/programmes undertaken by HAZs in relation to children and young people

Clinical focus	Behavioural focus	Structural/environmental focus
• Asthma prevention and treatment • Specialist child health services e.g. paediatric cardiology • Speech therapy services • Low birth-weight babies • Immunisation • Children with complex medical needs	• Teenage pregnancy • Sexual health • Healthy schools (behaviour focus) • Lifestyles – healthy eating, exercise • Sun safety projects • Smoking cessation • Mental health interventions • Breastfeeding • Oral health • Drug work, substance misuse • Youth crime • Proof-of-age scheme • Reducing accidents • Bullying work	• Healthy schools • Work with looked-after children, children at risk, young people leaving care • Links with Sure Start and Sure Start Plus • Links with Education Action Zones • Food initiatives – breakfast clubs, food co-ops • Rent Deposit Scheme • Mental health interventions • Youth crime • Including children and young people in planning and service delivery/youth forums • Links with SRB • Links with Home Start • Links with New Deal for Communities

themselves were complex entities operating in what has been described as the increasingly complex open system of health and health care (Plesk and Greenhalgh 2001; Plesk and Wilson 2001). Key factors that contributed to policy change included:

- early pressures
- planning and performance management
- ministerial priorities
- budgets.

Early pressures

HAZs were launched with a great deal of enthusiasm. At the national level they were described as leading the way in addressing health inequalities after years of relative neglect. At the local level the emphasis on partnership and community involvement was particularly welcomed, as was the relative freedom offered to HAZs to determine their own priorities for action. In the first round of interviews with HAZ project managers in first wave zones, there was a real sense that HAZs represented a new and promising approach to addressing long standing problems in deprived communities (Judge et al. 1999). Local evaluations conducted in individual HAZs reported similar levels of enthusiasm during the early years of the initiative (Sullivan et al. 1999; Crawshaw et al. 2002).

This initial enthusiasm was tempered with concerns about a number of aspects of the HAZ agenda. First, there was widespread recognition that the objectives set out for HAZs were extremely challenging. Even with the promise of a seven-year lifespan, a great deal was expected from Health Action Zones, as one project manager explained:

> HAZ is incredibly ambitious, incredibly ambitious. I mean it involves a paradigm shift in terms of how health and social care are delivered, and thought about. Seven years is nowhere [near] long enough, [we] are at the very beginning of that process. It is a fundamental, cultural, attitudinal change in terms of institutions and how they relate with each other.

Coupled with this recognition regarding the scale of the task facing HAZs was considerable scepticism about the amount of funding available. Commentators pointed out that the available funding was relatively trivial compared with spending on mainstream services, and that these resources would be an insufficient incentive to overcome entrenched differences between local organisations (Higgins 1998; Shaw et al. 1999). Project managers themselves recognised that resources were limited:

> We are actually talking about a small pot of money. Therefore what we are using the HAZ money to do is to look at a different way of spending and prioritising through joint working. It is very much about facilitating existing agencies to spend their own money differently.

Resources were a challenge for HAZs both in terms of the level of funding and the way in which it was administered by central government. The overall level of resource meant that infrastructure consisted of a small number of HAZ-funded staff. These staff were then reliant upon input from a range of other actors employed by partner organisations who gave their time on a voluntary basis. The HAZ effectively relied on the goodwill of partner agencies – and this goodwill varied depending on local circumstances and stage of development. As other research has identified, this situation was exacerbated by the existence of other area-based initiatives operating in the same locations as HAZs, with similar expectations regarding partnership working and similar levels of available resource (DETR 2002).

The manner in which funds were made available to HAZs also posed challenges for the initiative. Despite the promise of a seven-year lifespan, in practice funds were made available on a yearly basis through annual allocations to health authorities. This meant that projects funded directly from HAZ monies were relatively short term. This provided opportunities as well as constraints. The intention was always for HAZs to trial new ways of working and then encourage partner agencies to mainstream successful interventions. The value of investing in innovative interventions was emphasised, at least in the early years of HAZs, and as a result many areas did experiment with new approaches (Benzeval and Meth 2002a). However, the short-term nature of available funds posed problems in terms of staffing projects and evaluating their achievements (Bauld et al. 2002).

An additional early pressure for HAZs was the need to demonstrate results relatively quickly. In part because of the initially high profile ascribed to HAZs, project managers reported that there was pressure to demonstrate what the HAZ was achieving at a time when projects and programmes were still being established. Sullivan and colleagues (2003a) have described this as a consequence of the political cycle, with government unwilling to wait for new policy interventions to 'bed down' before demanding evidence of impact. One of the consequences of this demand for tangible 'evidence' of progress was that HAZ partnerships placed an early emphasis on recording outputs from individual projects rather than taking the time to consider how best to structure their activities to realise longer term outcomes.

Planning and performance management

Originally, HAZs were encouraged to develop local solutions to local health problems through the development of bids and subsequently, implementation plans (Powell and Moon 2001). As the guidance for HAZs stated (DH 1997a):

> The purpose of HAZs would be to bring together all those contributing to the health of the local population to develop and implement a locally agreed strategy for improving the health of local people ... The creation of HAZs is intended to release local energy and innovation.
>
> (DH 1997a, p. 3)

The result of this early encouragement of diversity was a huge variety of intended projects and programmes, as we outlined earlier. Details of these activities were included in annual implementation plans. These were described by a senior civil servant as 'living documents, updated as the HAZ moves forward particularly in the programme detail but also in work with communities'. HAZs were required to include a number of elements in these plans, including a vision statement, an environmental assessment and an overview of programme targets. In addition they explained how HAZs would involve partner agencies, plan local evaluation and put in place governance arrangements.

An early review of HAZ implementation plans revealed a gap between the longer term aspirations of HAZs and the projects they had chosen to invest in (Judge 2000). HAZ stakeholders identified the local problems that they wished to address, and what they wanted to achieve in terms of health improvement and tackling inequalities. However, the step that proved extremely difficult for HAZs was articulating how specific activities would achieve particular intermediate outcomes that would in turn contribute to the realisation of the long-term goals. To a certain degree, linking up problems, intermediate outcomes and longer term goals remained a challenge for HAZs throughout their lifetime, but in the early days of the initiative it was particularly marked. This problem is not unique to HAZs; instead it is a common characteristic of complex community-based initiatives (Connell et al. 1995; Fulbright-Anderson et al. 1998). A lack of robust and convincing local plans can contribute to an 'implementation gap' between the aspirations of central government and what local agencies are then able to put in place on the ground (Exworthy et al. 2000).

The difficulty that HAZs encountered in developing convincing plans posed problems for central government, who were eager to see results from investment at the earliest opportunity. Early attempts by the Department of Health to monitor HAZ progress through the usual channels (primarily financial) were deemed unsatisfactory, and a decision was taken to invest in a new system of monitoring, as a senior civil servant explained:

> The problem was that the reporting structures we had just didn't deliver information that was of any use to us. It told us how they were spending money but they didn't tell us what they were achieving with it very well.

In an attempt to better understand the types of activities that HAZs were investing in, as well as any outputs or outcomes, a performance management system was introduced in 1999. While the approach involved was similar to the reporting mechanisms imposed on other parts of the health service and local government, the specific framework that was eventually agreed was unique to HAZs. It involved the production of 'high-level statement' documentation on a quarterly basis. Each statement included targets that the HAZ hoped to achieve (such as reducing teenage pregnancy rates by 10 per cent in five years) and illustrated how particular activities contributed to the achievement of these goals. High-level statements, along with financial returns, were forwarded by HAZs to the Department of Health's regional offices, who were responsible for assessing the zones in their area twice yearly and using this information to report to ministers.

From 2000 onwards, the performance management information produced by HAZs was used to rate the zones' performance in relation to 'traffic lights' used across the NHS (DH 2000c). Most HAZs received a 'green' traffic light in repeated rounds of assessment but several zones were awarded 'red' status at different intervals and were subsequently encouraged to improve their performance or lose funding.

Despite a recognition amongst HAZ project managers of the value of careful planning and the need for accountability mechanisms, the scope and nature of high-level statements was heavily criticised for a number of reasons. First, the completion of these quarterly statements was difficult and time-consuming. As one project manager reported:

> They appear to have been developed by a mad man designed to make people on the ground go crazy, trying to fill them in. It feels like that the more the centre have tried to refine, the less clear in their purpose they've become.

In addition, project managers felt that the linear format of the statements did not accurately portray HAZ activities. As one interviewee stated: 'performance management is not a by-product of what we do, it doesn't fully reflect what we do – it's a separate system'. There was particular concern that the building of partnerships and work with communities that HAZs were conducting was not adequately captured or recognised within the high-level statement format. There was also some frustration that partner agencies, including other parts of the health system, had parallel but incompatible reporting requirements. This concern was not unique to HAZ: other studies of policy initiatives in the late 1990s identified a fundamental contradiction between the government's discourse of 'horizontal' partnership working on the one hand, and 'vertical' performance management systems on the other (Clarence and Painter 1998; Powell 1999).

Ministerial priorities

In October 1999, a new Secretary of State for Health, Alan Milburn, took up his position. Milburn introduced a number of significant reforms into the health service. He was particularly determined that the constituent parts of the NHS should work together to tackle leading causes of death such as heart disease and cancer, as well as addressing long-standing problems such as waiting times for treatment.

Milburn's view of what HAZs should be achieving differed from his predecessor, Frank Dobson. A senior civil servant explained:

> I think that Alan Milburn and Frank Dobson have quite different views and expectations ... whilst Frank Dobson was secretary of state he was incredibly keen and interested in health improvement. When we had Alan Milburn back he came with a very clear view of what he had to achieve, which was basically to save the NHS. He didn't see, I think, how HAZ contributed towards that. He felt that they had gone off into Tessa Jowell [Minister for Public Health] country.

Milburn's intention was to 'modernise' the NHS, an exercise that involved ensuring that all parts of the health service worked towards achieving key common objectives (Crawshaw et al. 2002). This meant that he was less willing to allow HAZs to continue addressing a wide range of locally determined issues. Instead he wanted them to focus on national priorities. As he reported to the Health Select Committee on Public Expenditure (House of Commons, 2002):

> We changed the regime so there is actually much tighter monitoring of the HAZs now. What I want them to do is to spend the majority of the resources that they get, which are quite considerable, on precisely the areas that we know will make the greatest difference, on dealing with CHD [Coronary Heart Disease], on improving cancer outcomes.

This change in ministerial expectations had significant implications for HAZs. They were told to modify their programmes and demonstrate how they were contributing to addressing CHD, cancer, mental health and other NHS priorities. For some zones this involved only minor changes to their programme. For others the shift was more significant. Almost all project managers (twenty-five out of twenty-six), when interviewed in the autumn of 2000, pointed to ministerial priorities as a significant cause of a shift in direction for their HAZ. For all HAZs, it was clear that their original remit of developing local solutions to address local health problems had changed.

With the benefit of hindsight, this shift in priorities heralded the end of the initial enthusiasm and optimism that had characterised HAZs. The profile of the initiative, at least at the national level, began to lessen. Milburn's agenda for the NHS meant that the objectives of HAZs changed significantly, and thus their energies had to be directed towards a new set of priorities. Other studies have demonstrated that policy success is usually related to clear and consistent objectives (Exworthy et al. 2000; Wismar and Busse 2002). Thus when the goals of HAZs changed, their capacity to demonstrate impact – both in relation to their original objectives and the revised HAZ agenda – was also undermined.

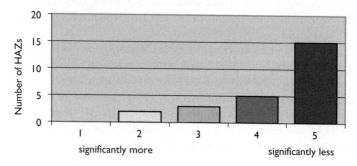

Figure 4.2 Comparison of total budgetary allocation for HAZs for 2000/01 with what they originally expected to spend that year

Budgets

Unease surrounding the shift in ministerial priorities was exacerbated in the spring of 2001 by a reduction in the level of resource available to HAZs (Hansard 2000a). This arose, at least in part, because a number of HAZs had underspent in 1999/2000, to the tune of £23 million in total (Hansard 2000b). This had arisen because of the slow development of particular programmes and problems such as difficulties recruiting staff. Indeed in interviews in 2000, eighteen project managers reported dissatisfaction with the availability of skilled and trained staff at an operational level. The reduction of the 2000/01 budget affected most zones. For example, South Yorkshire Coalfields experienced a £789,000 cut to their annual budget. Figure 4.2 illustrates the extent to which project managers felt that their budgetary allocation for 2000/01 represented more or less than the amount they had been expecting.

As Figure 4.2 illustrates, the vast majority of project managers reported that their 2000/01 budget amounted to fewer resources than they had been expecting. Just two project managers indicated that the allocation represented an increase, in both cases because, although the core budget was reduced, other sources of funds were available (such as smoking, drugs and innovations funding), which raised the overall level of resource.

Project managers subsequently highlighted the difficulty of managing these cuts, the impact of which was more than financial. Exacerbated by press stories outlining the budget changes, they expressed frustration about the way in which these had been determined and communicated to HAZs. As one project manager said:

> The budget cuts added to a sense of loss of confidence in HAZs nationally; it damaged community relations.

HAZs adopted varied strategies to deal with the budget cuts and resulting problems. Some reduced the number of programmes, as one project manager explained:

> [The] main programme reduced. We stopped the transport and health programme and the community-based initiative on mental health. We delayed the low birth weight and intensive case management in primary care programme.

Other project managers reported that changes to the budget did not significantly affect the work programme, because they were able to call on the resources of partner organisations to support various projects:

> [We had] 25 per cent less core budget, however more money [was] coming from other sources. [We] managed the risk by cross-funding projects.

Others decided not to invest in forthcoming activities, and expressed anxiety about the future:

> We managed this year, but we're very concerned about next year, we need more next year. If we don't we will have to make people redundant and stop programmes. We cannot make further investments, which will stifle the programme next year.

Concern about future funding is a common issue for initiatives with a time-limited lifespan and in this respect the views of project managers echo those of staff from other initiatives (DETR 2000a; Bauld et al. 2005). The budget cuts of 2001 did, however, exacerbate these concerns. The cuts were perceived as representing a loss of central government confidence in HAZs. This in turn affected the zones locally, as it caused some partner agencies to reconsider their level of commitment. In an environment of many and competing policy initiatives, most of which relied upon the goodwill of local voluntary and community groups to function, HAZs began to be perceived as less important.

Neighbourhood renewal and NHS reform

Health Action Zones were the product of the first term of a new Labour government, as outlined in Chapter 1. As the government approached the election of 2001 and the possibility of a second term, there was an opportunity to take stock and determine whether the approach taken to public service reform was the right one. It was during this period that a new series of policies emerged, involving significant structural and organisational change for the NHS and local government. These changes were to provide both challenges and opportunities for HAZs, and ultimately to herald the end of the initiative.

New Labour's enthusiasm for area-based initiatives was one kind of policy that came under increasing scrutiny. By 2001 there was significant evidence from a range of sources that the plethora of ABIs was proving to be problematic. Reviewing regeneration initiatives, the Audit Commission commented:

> Our research indicates a growing local appetite for a rationalisation of the number of special and area-based initiatives. The current system poses a range of practical problems. Not only is it very complex, but ... agencies feel obliged to respond to the launching of initiatives with different criteria, planning cycles, objectives, geographical coverage and reporting and evaluation arrangements.
>
> (Audit Commission 2002, p. 16)

Some parts of England had become host to a large number of overlapping ABIs, causing duplication and other problems highlighted in the DETR-funded evaluation of collaboration and coordination between ABIs (DETR 2002). Reviews of the evidence questioned whether area-based approaches were in fact the best way to assist the most deprived households (DETR 2000c). At the same time, extensive research into the causes and nature of social exclusion in Britain culminated in the recognition that a new approach to reviving 'failing' communities was required. The result was the development of a national strategy for neighbourhood renewal, launched in 2001 (Social Exclusion Unit 2001). The strategy aimed to develop a more integrated way to reducing a range of inequalities across England's most deprived communities. At the heart of the strategy was the development of Local Strategic Partnerships (DETR, 2001). These bodies, led by local government, were intended to consolidate existing partnership structures, including HAZs. The intention to bring HAZs within the LSP umbrella was first outlined in the *NHS Plan*, which stated:

> The NHS will help develop Local Strategic Partnerships, into which, in the medium term, health action zones and other local action zones could be integrated to strengthen links between health, education, employment and other causes of social exclusion.
>
> (DH 2000c, p. 111)

In addition to the changes heralded by neighbourhood renewal, HAZs were affected by reforms within the NHS in England. These structural changes were first outlined in the *NHS Plan* (DH 2000c) and subsequently developed in the document *Shifting the Balance of Power* (DH 2001d). They amounted to a complete restructuring of key components of the health service. Perhaps most significantly for HAZs, they included the abolition of health authorities (through which HAZ funding was originally distributed) and the creation of larger Strategic Health Authorities and, at the local level, the formation of Primary Care Groups (PCGs) and subsequently, Primary Care Trusts (PCTs). PCTs were to become the main commissioning and delivery arm of the health service, controlling 75 per cent of the NHS budget by 2004 (Doyle, 2001). In addition, they were to bear responsibility for addressing health inequalities, in partnership with LSPs. *Shifting the Balance of Power* stated that 'HAZs are to be reabsorbed with mainstream health funding through primary care trusts' (DH 2001d, p. 14).

Thus, by 2002, the structure of key partner organisations for HAZs was transformed. In addition, the abolition of health authorities raised questions about how future HAZ funding would be provided. Some of the anxiety surrounding this issue was relieved when an additional years funding was provided directly to HAZs from March 2002, but without the promise of any future resources. The evaluation explored the impact of all these changes including:

- future direction for HAZs
- Local Strategic Partnerships
- Primary Care Trusts.

Future direction for HAZs

The advent of LSPs and PCTs, and the clear intention to merge HAZ functions within these organisations, meant a shift in focus for those working within HAZs. Project managers were encouraged to focus their efforts on 'mainstreaming' projects and activities. This involved working with partner organisations to convince them to fund interventions that had initially been supported by HAZs. It also involved encouraging agencies – in particular LSPs and PCTs – to adopt HAZ 'ways of working', specifically models of partnership working and engaging communities. The process of mainstreaming is discussed in more detail in Chapter 6.

Mainstreaming provided HAZs with new opportunities, in that the emphasis was on influencing emerging organisations rather than focussing on delivery of projects. However, by 2002 it had become apparent to everyone involved with HAZs that events had overtaken the initiative and that the end was in sight. Project managers were asked whether they believed that HAZs would continue 'in their current form' after March 2002. Most felt positive about progress continuing at the local level, but were much less certain regarding the future direction of national policy in relation to HAZs. Project managers were generally less optimistic as time went on – responses to this question were less positive in late 2001 than in the previous year.

Although project managers recognised the potential of LSPs and PCTs to take forward the work of HAZ, they also expressed a significant amount of uncertainty about the future. This uncertainty was both personal and more general. Personal concerns were expressed in terms of where their skills and those of other HAZ staff would be deployed. More general uncertainty concerned the upheaval associated with significant organisational restructuring. There was also a recognition that if HAZs ceased to exist in their current form a number of benefits could be lost. These included:

- the loss of a unified health focus across the area the HAZ covered
- the dilution of health issues within broader partnerships with competing priorities
- the 'submergence' of HAZs into LSPs, relegating health to a less prominent position than other issues such as crime or education
- a potential loss of learning through short-termism.

It was not until January 2003 that HAZs received notification that PCTs would receive three years' funding from April 2003 to take forward the aims of the initiative. A letter from the DH (2003b) to project managers stated:

> In line with *Shifting the Balance of Power*, HAZ programmes should by now have become mainstreamed within local PCTs' priorities and activity. These PCTs will therefore be responsible for decisions about how new resources will be used. However, our expectation is that these decisions will continue to support the overall aims of the HAZ particularly on tackling health inequalities and therefore assist PCTs to deliver the national inequality targets within their areas.

At the time of writing, the legacy of HAZs remains unclear following the decision to channel HAZ funds through PCTs. No specific guidance has been given to PCTs on the allocation of these funds. Given the workload and financial pressures faced by PCTs in their early years, there is concern that the health improvement agenda will be overtaken by the 'must dos' of the acute sector such as dealing with hospital waiting lists and providing front-line medical services (Freeman 2002). In addition, by the time this new funding had been announced, a number of HAZ 'offices' had been disbanded. Full-time project managers and support staff had left, to be replaced by individuals within PCTs or Strategic Health Authorities who inherited a HAZ remit as just one part of their job. Lambeth, Southwark and Lewisham HAZ (2003), for instance, issued a final newsletter thanking partner organisations and community groups for their contribution and providing contact details for HAZ staff, who had all moved to new posts. Thus by April 2003, HAZs as separate entities with a clear identity had

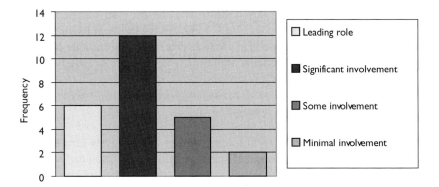

Figure 4.3 Level of involvement of HAZs in LSP development

effectively ceased to exist. It is thus worth examining how HAZ activities and ways of working were influencing LSPs and PCTs in the final stage of their lifespan, from the perspective of project managers.

Local Strategic Partnerships

The formation of local strategic partnerships began in 2001, and most HAZs made early efforts to become involved in their development. Project managers expressed optimism that LSPs had the potential to take forward the work of HAZs, either in terms of specific activities or ways of working. The clearest sense of optimism regarding the future of HAZ work within LSPs emerged in areas where the HAZ and LSP were to be coterminous.

In November 2001, project managers described the level of involvement of their HAZ in LSP development. Figure 4.3 outlines their responses.

As Figure 4.3 demonstrates, eighteen (69 per cent) project managers perceived the role of their HAZ in LSP development to be 'leading' or 'significant'. This role took a variety of forms, such as:

- individuals working within the HAZ adopting a leadership role in fledgling LSPs
- part-time posts in the regional government office established with HAZ funding specifically to influence LSP development
- HAZ project managers leading health subcommittees or programmes for one or more LSPs in their area.

By the spring of 2002, LSPs were at differing stages of development across England. For instance, multiple hierarchies were observed in areas where there was a county and several district councils. Some district councils had merged to form one LSP, but some had formed separate LSPs. Some HAZs with multiple levels of LSP described it as a 'nesting' structure. One area with this formation had devolved the HAZ budget to locality groups that formed the health groups on the district level LSPs. Simultaneously there was an overarching HAZ board, the aim of which was to put health 'on everyone's agenda'. The HAZ board linked with district-level LSPs and county-level LSPs. Some project managers working with multiple layers of LSP expressed concern, for example:

> I think the issue around LSPs is that they are a relatively new body and they're now sitting on top of existing structures. I think for a while there's going to be some conflict as to which body has the authority.

HAZs that had invested in partnership working with a wide range of organisations and enjoyed positive relationships with local government reported that these relationships were helping their role within LSPs. In these areas, project managers felt that they had valuable lessons to share:

> The cultural change involved in working with a range of stakeholders in a 'whole systems way' had been well developed by HAZ ... so [for us] it wasn't as much of a shock to the system as it might have been in some areas.

One project manager said that 'LSPs are based on a lot of the work that had already been established through the HAZ'. Thus in some areas, HAZ work was serving as a starting point for LSP development, either through the continuation of specific projects or the adoption of procedures or ways of working that were established by the HAZ.

Primary Care Trusts

In some areas the transition from health authorities to Strategic Health Authorities and PCTs was relatively smooth, with HA boundaries closely matching the new PCTs. In other areas the transition was more complex. The impact of these changes on Health Action Zones was not merely one of changing organisational accountability. There was also a great deal of diversity in the way in which HAZs 'fitted into' PCTs, the role they were adopting within these new organisations, and the extent to which positive lessons from HAZs were being transferred.

As with LSPs, project managers were asked about emerging relationships with PCTs in three sets of interviews. During the first round of PCT-relevant questions in the spring of 2001, all project managers indicated that they were engaged, on behalf of the HAZ, in trying to influence the development of PCTs in their area. Nineteen (73 per cent) project managers reported that their HAZ had very good or good relations with the (developing) PCTs in their area.

When discussing the HAZ–PCT relationships in their locality, project managers raised a number of issues regarding the opportunities and constraints they faced. These varied between areas, but many related to key themes such as the upheaval caused by reform, leadership, boundary issues and concerns regarding the priority of HAZ work within the PCT agenda. For instance, networks and contacts built up over time were dissolved, as one project manager explained:

> It has been disrupting in the sense that we had good working relationships between key players then suddenly the key players disappeared.

More significantly, HAZs themselves were 'dissolved' as staff moved to other organisations:

> Because of a lack of certainty all our staff disappeared at the end of March [2002] apart from myself, so I've had no infrastructure to continue our work.

In particular, the changes meant that key local leaders had moved on. Concerns were expressed that this was resulting in a loss of expertise in some HAZ areas, particularly regarding effective ways to address health inequalities locally.

Boundary issues with PCTs also proved to be a challenge in some areas. In some parts of England, this shift to PCTs meant more complex relationships, with the HAZ dealing with several PCTs rather than one or two HAs. This proved challenging not just for HAZs but their local partner organisations:

> The three PCTs are working co-operatively ... but it does mean that other players like the local authority are dealing with three organisations where they used to deal with one, which is bound to complicate life.

Finally, despite optimism that PCTs would be encouraged by central government to maintain a specific health inequalities remit and be provided with funds to tackle the issue, project managers were aware of the multiple demands on these new organisations and the risk that HAZ-related issues would be 'sidelined'. Competing priorities and financial concerns had implications for activities initially undertaken by HAZs. This meant that projects were terminated when attempts to convince a PCT to continue the work were unsuccessful. This was particularly the case with interventions that had a broad population health focus (such as drug prevention and emergency contraception projects, for example) rather than ones that fitted easily into a more medical model of service delivery.

Conclusion

The changes experienced by HAZs between their establishment in 1998 and their effective dismantling five years later are not unique. There are similarities with previous large-scale policy initiatives launched amid much enthusiasm, whose original aims and expectations became diluted as the reality of translating policy into practice took shape. HAZs were required to adapt as political imperatives altered; from an initial focus on bottom-up approaches to a more top-down agenda as the pressure to demonstrate progress heightened. They were affected by changes within central government (such as shifting ministerial priorities) and problems at the local level (such as a lack of capacity in relation to planning). Eventually they were superseded by significant structural reforms that meant that many of the organisations involved in designing and implementing HAZ programmes were redundant. Along the way, however, they invested in a range of innovative and important activities and processes that will be described in greater detail in the chapters that follow.

Chapter 5

Building capacity for collaboration

Helen Sullivan, Marian Barnes and Elizabeth Matka

Introduction

The national HAZ initiative sought to address a key cross-cutting policy problem, that of improving community health and reducing persistent health inequalities. Overcoming the challenges presented by such a complex policy problem required interventions that cut across the conventional boundaries of national and local governance and which could be realised only through the joint efforts of public authorities, the private sector, voluntary organisations and communities. HAZs were built upon the most familiar form of joint action, the multi-organisational partnership. 'A formal expression of shared commitment to act in the common interest', it is a way of 'sharing responsibility and overcoming the inflexibility created by organisational and even national boundaries' (Sullivan and Skelcher 2002, p. 1). Under New Labour, community participation in partnerships and the delivery of social programmes assumed great importance and this was reflected in the guidance for potential HAZs issues by the Department for Health.

As outlined in Chapter 2, neither partnership working nor community involvement were particularly new in UK public policy. In common with many other countries, the United Kingdom had developed a keen interest in the use of partnership mechanisms and service user involvement initiatives as part of the enthusiasm for *marketisation* that had taken hold in the latter decades of the twentieth century. However, despite this increasing incidence of cross-sector collaboration through partnership evident in the field of UK public policy, the capacity of the various stakeholders to take joint action remained questionable (Hall et al. 1996; Benyon and Edwards 1999; Hudson et al. 1999). Therefore, given the emphasis on using the national evaluation of HAZs as a tool for learning, this part of the HAZ evaluation centred on the experience of five HAZs in 'building capacity for collaboration' amongst organisational partners and with communities: Bradford and Sandwell – HAZs where the original configuration involved coterminous health and local authorities; Manchester, Salford and Trafford

(MaST) and Lambeth, Southwark and Lewisham (LSL) – 'complex' HAZs covering three local authorities and one or two health authority areas; and Northumberland, a predominantly rural HAZ including one health authority and two tiers of local government. Using a case study approach and working within the 'Theories of Change' framework, the evaluation followed the experiences of each of the five HAZs between 1999 and 2002, undertaking two rounds of interviews with key players, using postal questionnaires to obtain wider views on partnership working and community involvement in the HAZs, developing and employing a project reporting instrument to gain the views of sampled HAZ projects about partnership working and community involvement over time and attending and observing a variety of HAZ events and meetings (detailed discussions of our use of 'Theories of Change' are contained in Sullivan et al. 2002; Barnes, M. et al. 2003a).

The material presented in this chapter draws on this evaluation data to discuss three aspects of building capacity for collaboration: the strategies adopted by individual HAZs to promote collaboration and the influences on their development, the nature and degree of collaborative capacity generated in HAZs over their life time and the contribution of this collaborative capacity to the achievement of HAZ and other objectives.

Developing strategies for collaboration

Early HAZ strategies

In an early HAZ evaluation report four distinct approaches to local HAZ strategy development were identified: the consolidation strategy, mainstream strategy, emergent strategy and innovation strategy (Barnes et al. 2001). Importantly it was argued that,

> In view of the complexity and dynamic nature of HAZ activity, these [approaches] should be understood as a way of conceptualising strategies, rather than categorising HAZs. While it was possible to discern a dominant strand in each of the case studies, elements of these strategies appear in more than one HAZ.
>
> (Barnes et al. 2001, p. 14)

An examination of the experiences of the five case study HAZs serves to elaborate this point.

The consolidation strategy

This strategy was focused upon taking stock of progress already made within a HAZ area and finding ways of securing and building upon that progress. The underlying rationale for this approach was that the problems and desired outcomes were well known and agreed locally, that past activities demonstrated some capacity to achieve these outcomes and that the purpose of HAZ was to facilitate further progress by removing any existing obstacles and opening up new opportunities.

The work of Sandwell HAZ best exemplified this strategy. Here the HAZ was used to 'add value' to existing work wherever possible and to develop new streams of work where these fitted with existing priorities. Ten programme areas were initially established to work in this way. A key programme area was the 'public information and community involvement' (PICCI) programme that sought to build an infrastructure for public information and communication as well as to facilitate community involvement by working through communities of geography and identity, the organised community and voluntary sectors and through community development officers within the borough. The governance of the HAZ was likewise through an existing mechanism – the Health Partnership – an arm of the borough's strategic civic partnership.

Northumberland HAZ also manifested elements of a consolidation strategy. This was derived from the county's strong reputation in relation to the joint work undertaken between health and social services. The HAZ provided an opportunity to consolidate this work.

The mainstream strategy

This strategy was concerned with using HAZ to secure mainstream change so that all organisations and sectors better understood how they could contribute to improved health. The underlying rationale for this strategy was of health as a cross-cutting issue that all sectors had a role in promoting. These roles were not always well understood and the HAZ was seen as a powerful catalyst for change which needed to be embedded in longer term policy and delivery processes.

The Bradford HAZ programme was closest to this kind of strategy. The emphasis on using HAZ to support infrastructure change and development to take forward a more 'joined-up' agenda in relation to health was clear in the Implementation Plan. This manifested itself in a number of ways: the focus on collaboration at all levels from front-line (through primary care groups) to strategy (through the Health Improvement Plan); the establishment of a community involvement team to link existing community activity with new opportunities for involvement; and the development of a comprehensive local evaluation programme to monitor and report on progress towards change. The governance of the HAZ also reflected this focus on mainstream change. The HAZ Partnership Board was closely linked to the pre-existing strategic body for the district – the Bradford Congress – and the Board itself sought wide cross-sectoral representation to engender a deeper and wider understanding of health.

Northumberland HAZ also exhibited elements of a mainstream strategy. The health/social services relationship though critical (see p. 89) was only one aspect of the Northumberland HAZ. The HAZ also sought to promote health as a cross-cutting issue, one that required an holistic approach involving all stakeholders. Hence the role of the HAZ was also to prioritise areas where mainstream change could be made and to use the HAZ to support partners and citizens in better understanding their role in achieving this change. Members of the public were seen to have a vital role to play in the delivery of this strategy. Community empowerment was identified as a core principle of Northumberland HAZ and a separate workstream established to pursue this objective.

The emergent strategy

The emphasis of this strategy was to find the best way to deliver positive change in health improvement and health inequality in a complex and somewhat unfamiliar environment. The underlying rationale for this strategy was that the HAZ entity was an artificial creation and therefore the wholesale application of a single strategy may be inappropriate and counterproductive. Here the particular needs and dynamics of the constituent parts of the HAZ were acknowledged to require the application of different approaches. Nonetheless opportunities for HAZ-wide endeavour to complement local activity were explored. At the same time, the HAZ offered opportunities to test out new ways of doing things in specific service areas in order to establish 'good practice' across the HAZ.

The activities of MaST HAZ illustrated the operation of this strategy in practice. Initial attempts to work in a client-based HAZ-wide manner proved difficult in part because of the need to establish HAZ-wide systems and processes to facilitate working across such a large and complex area. While ultimately unsustainable, this initial experience provided the HAZ with evidence about how it could best maximise its zone status.

It subsequently set about working in a more targeted manner, within 'Development Sites' in local authority areas and through 'trail blazing' policy or service specific initiatives. In both cases opportunities for learning through change were emphasised. In the case of Development Sites there were opportunities to consider how the HAZ could provide 'added value' to existing area-based regeneration, while in the case of policy or service activity, the emphasis was upon establishing 'what worked and why'. A number of programmes did operate across the zone but they were applied flexibly to meet different local circumstances. A centrally important programme that followed this pattern was the Community Programme which worked with communities in a variety of ways including as individual citizens, as groups of users or whole communities, as representatives or members of organisations and as contributors to decision making.

The governance arrangements for partnership in the HAZ followed a similar pattern with initial attempts to develop an all-embracing framework being replaced by a more streamlined partnership board with considerable devolution to the operational levels.

The innovation strategy

This strategy focused on a particular aspect of the HAZ agenda – innovation – and used it as an opportunity to challenge conventional approaches. The rationale underlying this strategy was that in order to genuinely transform prevailing policy and practices a widespread surge of innovation was needed to establish momentum for change and to test out a variety of new approaches.

LSL's HAZ strategy exemplified an attempt to develop and apply a strategy oriented toward innovation. Their Implementation Plan 'Children First' emphasised the need to focus on preventative work with children and families in order to secure the necessary changes in service provision, access and use to facilitate improved life chances among children in the three boroughs. Eight programme objectives were identified, all pertaining to children, families and/or young people. Delivery of these objectives was through working in partnership to create whole systems change and by listening to and working with communities. The governance arrangements for the HAZ tried to reflect this emphasis on innovation by specifying a key role for cross-organisational Programme Groups (existing below the HAZ Partnership Board and alongside the Executive Group) to commission projects in line with the principles of 'Children First'. These groups were replaced by 'learning networks' early on in the life of the HAZ. The role of the learning networks was to foster and spread good practice emerging from HAZ to relevant networks of professionals and others who were not in direct contact with HAZ but would be instrumental in sustaining progress made over the lifetime of the HAZ initiative.

Changing strategies for changing times

In each case the HAZ strategy that initially emerged was shaped by the prevailing local context. The extent to which the HAZ strategies changed over time depended upon the experience of implementation and the dynamics of the national agenda. Amongst the five case studies it was possible to distinguish those where there was significant change in strategy from those where the overall approach remained consistent over the life of the HAZ (see Table 5.1 for a summary). Crudely this differentiated the 'simple' HAZs from those working across multiple boundaries. In the latter a 'learning by

Table 5.1 The phases of HAZ

MaST	LSL	Sandwell	Bradford	Northumberland
Euphoria Building the infrastructure, spending the money, loss of direction.	Awareness of the size of the task and government pressure to spend money quickly. Scattergun creation of projects – 'chaotic and not thought through'. HAZ a series of projects rather than collective enterprise.	Establishment – developing plans already in place, catalysing change. Frantic time.	Waiting, anticipating – capitalising on shared concerns articulated pre-HAZ. Manic phase, lots of energy.	Establishment – building on existing partnership. Focus on structures and processes.
Revamping and revitalising following internal review. Establishing an identity but also some crises.	Internal review, leading to emphasis on whole systems change. Challenge of 'institutional racism' criticism met positively. Low point following change in national priorities. Devolution of delivery responsibility. HAZ as facilitator/ adviser.	Operational – carrying forward original plan with no major change in strategy. Dealing with a change in context – responding to changed national view of HAZ; the significance of possible new partners (PCG/Ts); funding uncertainty.	Time consumed by allocation of money. Concern about 'projectitis' tempered by mainstream change strategy. Frustration and disappointment at curtailment of seven-year programme.	Implementation – slight reconfiguration of programmes in the context of a stable strategy – emphasis on mainstream.
Impact of changes at the centre – 'drawn back to the NHS agenda'. Uncertainty and pessimism but also recommitment to local strategy and strengthening of internal identity.		Transitional – hiatus: 'eyes off the ball'. Impact of HA abolition. Coping with significant personnel change.	Reappraising and revisiting original priorities, reassertion of mainstream strategy.	Responding to changes in national emphasis – incorporation the 'must dos'. Funding uncertainty and insecurity.
Anticipating end of HAZ funding, consolidation and mainstreaming.	Following through process of devolution/ mainstreaming.	Future – principles to be taken forward outwith HAZ – 'the	Shifting the balance and losing our balance – break-up of HA destabilising. HAZ more marginal – questioning mainstream strategy.	Changing approach – a new style of leadership and greater informality. From the HAZ to the Care Trust. HAZ philosophy and

Table 5.1 The phases of HAZ (continued)

MaST	LSL	Sandwell	Bradford	Northumberland
A future beyond HAZ in selected areas. A less certain future at strategic level.	Developmental commissioning, dissemination of learning. Limitations due to lack of fit between local and national priorities. Uncertain role for HAZ in future.	concept not the label'. Setting down, aims being reasserted in a new context.	Joining up across new boundaries. New relationships forged. New opportunities for linking HAZ with mainstream – LSP and NRF.	commitment taken forward in a new guise.

Source: Barnes, M. et al. (2003b)

doing' process was essential prior to the determination of a sustainable strategy. So in MaST the original attempt to work across the whole HAZ proved unsustainable, while in LSL the attempt to catalyse innovation and broad-based change by funding a variety of projects (the 'scatter gun' approach) was limited by the failure to engage a wide enough variety of partners and community stakeholders in the process. In neither case did respondents think that the initial phases of work could be considered genuinely strategic, although in both cases, they were considered inevitable given the context, and important for their contribution to subsequent developments.

Changes in strategies also resulted from external pressures – both MaST and LSL broadened their original focus from an emphasis on children and young people in order to respond to a requirement that HAZs address national priorities. Elsewhere changes to strategies were more an issue of adjustments, although all needed to bring forward the development of succession strategies in view of the uncertainty about the long-term future of HAZ that set in midway through the programme. This was probably most clearly delineated in Northumberland HAZ where the HAZ moved quickly to establish a Care Trust (a new type of service delivery organisation that integrated health and social care functions) for the county, harking back to the strong health/social services relationship that had underpinned it. The LSP agenda also had a profound effect on the way in which HAZs planned for the future, reorienting HAZ perspectives on the contribution of health to local community strategies and influencing the way HAZs worked in relation to neighbourhood based initiatives such as neighbourhood renewal.

The preceding discussion has demonstrated the ways in which HAZ strategies both shaped and were shaped by the prevailing contexts in their attempts to facilitate collaboration. Implicit in the above is the suggestion that such strategies are multidimensional, incorporating the generation of collaborative capacity within and between individuals and organisations in addition to being present within the infrastructure of the collaboration itself. So far the discussion has centred upon the external manifestation of collaborative capacity; how HAZ strategies resulted in tangible collaborative endeavour. However, as already indicated, building collaborative capacity requires that individuals and organisations develop characteristics and orientations supportive of such endeavour. These traits and their manifestation in HAZ are discussed below.

The components of collaborative capacity

Sullivan and Skelcher (2002) provide a framework for examining collaborative capacity that is multidimensional and draws on a range of research to identify key components of collaborative capacity. In brief they argue that the generation of collaborative capacity amongst individuals requires the demonstration of particular *leadership* and *boundary spanning* skills to cata- lyse and sustain collaborative action. It also relies upon the existence of strong *trust* relationships between individuals. Finally the development and demonstration of the skills and attributes of individual collaborative capacity needs to be considered worthwhile by individuals, i.e. there has to be some kind of '*fit*' between the investment in collaborative capacity and the pre- vailing environment or context. At organisational level collaborative capac- ity also needs to be demonstrated through *organisational leadership* and *inter-organisational trust.* However, to achieve this requires other attrib- utes to be in place, specifically a *collaborative organisational culture* and an orientation towards *learning.*

Each of these features is explored in the context of HAZ in the following sections.

Individual capacity

Leadership

In recent years considerable attention has been paid to the role of leadership in the transformation of public services. Sullivan and Skelcher (2002) argue that while leadership is central to collaboration, traditional approaches to leadership that focus on the role of the formally designated leader whom others follow are inappropriate to a collaborative environment where leader- ship is multiple and possibly contested. In such an environment greater cre- dence is attached to the personal authority an individual can command rather than their formal organisational position. This suggests a greater reliance on the possession of personal attributes that engender this author- ity. For Luke (1997) these attributes are contained within individuals who display what he describes as 'catalytic leadership' comprising certain core skills: the capacity to think and act strategically, the application of interper- sonal skills to relate to and successfully motivate others, an ability to focus on results and the possession of personal integrity that is acknowledged by others.

These core skills and the 'catalytic leadership' capacity that they generated were much in evidence and also highly regarded in the HAZ case studies. In some instances the very existence, character and/or success of the HAZ was closely identified with single individuals. Elsewhere the emphasis on 'cat- alytic leadership' was just as strong but it was associated with the activities and commitment of a group of people within the HAZ.

Leadership capacity emerged in different ways and in different locations in HAZ. For some the HAZ initiative represented an opportunity to use existing skills and capacities in the pursuit of shared goals. Here HAZ was a vehicle or conduit for pre-existing capacity. For others HAZ represented an opportunity for personal growth, to develop new skills or capacities through taking a leadership role in HAZ or to test out the utilities of existing skills and capacities in an entirely new partnership environment. For the most part opportunities for personal growth were identified and taken up by individuals themselves. However in some cases a capacity 'gap' within the HAZ was identified and a specific individual identified and sought out to fill it. For example in MaST HAZ a putative 'community leader' was identified within a targeted neighbourhood who subsequently became a key figure in the local delivery of the HAZ programme.

An important feature of HAZ was the sense of 'permission' to act differently that participants experienced. This was evident in all of the case study HAZs and extended beyond HAZ leaders. However, this notion of 'permission' was particularly important for those in leadership roles, as it meant not only that they could operate differently but also that they too could give permission to others in their organisations/sectors to do likewise.

While the core components of 'catalytic leadership' underpinned the activities of HAZ leaders, the style and emphasis varied between and within HAZs over time. In some cases this change of emphasis was managed within the existing leadership group, with individuals taking on different roles. However, in most cases the change of emphasis coincided with or was precipitated by the loss of a key leader to a role outside the HAZ. In Northumberland where the HAZ had devolved considerable power and responsibility to programmes, the loss of the key leader was seen as an opportunity to reshape the leadership of the initiative in the implementation phase. Key figures in the HAZ retained their role as HAZ 'champions' while a newly appointed Director of Public Health was given oversight of the running of the whole programme. In a similar situation in MaST HAZ the loss of the HAZ leader at the point at which the HAZ initiative was beginning to move out of implementation towards exit and the familiar partnership structures were in a state of flux, meant that there was a need for a HAZ leader who could manage this transition whilst retaining the coherence of HAZ potentially single-handed.

Whilst a change in the style and embodiment of leadership was sometimes valuable or necessary as HAZs evolved, in some cases a loss of significant individuals in leadership roles had a destabilising effect. Such losses were, in part, a consequence of the centrally imposed rule changes that we have discussed elsewhere (Barnes, M. et al. 2003a; see also Chapter 4 in this book).

All of the case study HAZs contained clearly identified 'community involvement champions' amongst their leaders. However, the success of the HAZ in developing a programme that was able to work with and take account of community perspectives appears to be linked to the centrality of the 'community involvement champion' to the HAZ initiative. So for example in MaST and Bradford where the HAZ directors were identified as 'catalytic leaders' with a personal understanding and passion for community involvement, the HAZ was publicly imbued with a community ethos. In Northumberland the closer association of the HAZ leader with strategic management and delivery meant that it was harder to locate the community orientation despite the high personal credibility of the public involvement programme manager.

Another difference in leadership style noted within the case studies was the emphasis given to building-in redundancy. While all the case studies contained leaders that were able to motivate others to act, some were self consciously attempting to increase the capacity for self-sufficiency amongst staff knowing that their tenure (and that of HAZ) was limited. For others the emphasis appeared to be on retaining key individual leaders for as long as possible so as to maintain the motivational ethos they provided.

Reticulists

Leadership was not sufficient of itself. As important were the skills and attributes of those who acted as 'reticulists or boundary spanners' at all levels in the HAZ. Sullivan and Skelcher (2002) characterise boundary spanners or reticulists as: skilled communicators with excellent networking skills enabling them to gain entry to a variety of settings; empathetic individuals who are able to understand a situation from a variety of perspectives, making them good negotiators and also appreciative of the constraints that other operate under; and creative people who are able to think laterally to solve problems. Reticulists or boundary-spanners are able to play a variety of roles in collaborations to facilitate action amongst others.

As in the case of HAZ leaders, there is evidence in the case study HAZs of reticulists perceiving HAZ as a route for applying their skills and of others seeking to make use of HAZ as an opportunity to develop such skills. The most commonly articulated capacities of reticulists cited in the case studies were networking, creativity, co-ordination, problem solving and communication. Those most obviously identified as reticulists were those whose job it was to 'add value' to action on the ground, usually with a specific community involvement/development focus. The Community Involvement workers at the PCG/PCTs in Bradford, the Healthy Living Development Managers in Northumberland, and the Community Development Coordinators in LSL all fulfilled this role. However, while these contributions were critical in achieving HAZ objectives, this was not the only level at which reticulists operated. So in Bradford the Health Partnerships manager played this role at a strategic level as did the Director of Public Health in Sandwell.

For reticulists the sense of 'permission' provided by HAZ was vitally important in legitimising their activities and helping to provide a 'fertile context' as it was expressed in one HAZ. While reticulists will deploy their skills and capacities wherever they can, it is much easier to do so in a sympathetic environment such as the one HAZ provided at least initially. In some cases expectations about the degree of freedom that HAZ would offer to work in innovative and risky ways were frustrated by the requirement to deliver on centrally defined priorities and objectives. What also remains uncertain from the evaluation is the extent to which the experience of HAZ facilitated change amongst non-enthusiasts about the potential value and contribution of those with reticulist capacities.

Trust

Sullivan and Skelcher (2002) argue that trust is a key component in collaboration and is particularly important in the individually based informal networks that underpin formal partnerships. The literature on trust relationships between individuals reveals a number of common themes associated with building and maintaining trust including reputation, competence, reliability, altruism, shared codes of conduct and the dynamics of trust. This last is particularly important in collaborative relationships as it draws attention to the fact that trust may be developed and lost in the process of collaborating (Mayer et al. 1995; Jones and George 1998; Lane and Bachmann 1998; Rousseau et al. 1998). Mayer et al. (1995) emphasise that the development of trust between individuals is based upon a combination of personal and professional attributes, for example combining a technical ability to do the job with altruistic motivations and individual integrity. Maintaining trust relationships over time requires the demonstration of reliability and dependability in relation to these attributes (Jones and George 1998; Rousseau et al. 1998).

These aspects of trust resonated with the case studies. For HAZ staff particularly, the ability to demonstrate their competence to other stakeholders was key to building trust, although it worked both ways, as in Bradford where the pre-existing area co-ordinators and the HAZ community involvement workers had many shared interests. For the area co-ordinators it was not only important that they were confident in the competence of the HAZ staff, but also necessary to demonstrate their own competence to these staff. This was accomplished by offering to organise and co-facilitate a community event. The success of this helped to build trust between the relevant individuals and led to further deeper collaboration. The impact of success as a spur to consolidate trust relationships was echoed in Northumberland where the importance of building trust through joint action (as opposed to building trust to facilitate it) was emphasised. Stakeholders in Northumberland were also keen to highlight the power of trust, emphasising that trust relationships last beyond individual roles or jobs and that once trust is built collaborative action can be sustained through informal rather than formal mechanisms.

However, one important aspect of trust – the absence of it and the conditions for fostering it – was also highlighted by the case study work. The absence of trust was cited in circumstances where individuals found themselves in unfamiliar partnerships with people they had little experience of and with organisations to which theirs might be antithetical. Personality clashes were also cited as both reasons for and the result of an absence of trust. These circumstances were most apparent in those HAZs that might be considered 'artificial' creations, where there was little shared experience and the decision to join together may have been rather forced. In such circumstances one HAZ – MaST – adopted a proactive stance, seeking to surface and confront differences and tensions between individuals, particularly amongst the strategic partners. For a time the HAZ employed a consultant to observe and work with the strategic partners to build the partnership and in so doing address latent conflicts. In addition the HAZ frequently faced media attention and criticism due to some of the more risky projects that it sponsored, such as an emergency contraception scheme. The need to provide a 'united front' in such a critical environment and particularly the need to provide support and protection for the staff delivering these 'risky' projects meant that the HAZ partnership was forced to reflect on the extent to which its members had shared values and aspirations and this in turn helped to generate trust through shared action.

Barnes and Prior (1996, 1998) discuss the significance of trust in renewing relationships between public services and their users. Fundamental to this is the notion of *reciprocal* trust – if citizens and service users are to have trust in public services, service providers must demonstrate trust in them. The relevance of this in the context of the discussion of the development of collaborative capacity is that it draws attention to ways in which HAZs may have created opportunities for service providers to become more trusting of users and communities, as well as vice versa. There are examples of this in HAZ, even if the purposes of action were not expressed in this way. Thus apparently 'risky' projects involving young men on the verge of criminal activity acting as mentors to others, giving teenagers more power to take control over their sexuality, or enabling mental health service users to find ways of dealing with their problems outside the medical model, can all be considered examples of ways of working which can build reciprocal trust. In a different way, enabling community members to take on significant leadership roles: chairing groups, deciding on the allocation of grants, and running community projects, are indicative of a greater preparedness on the part of 'officials' to trust 'the public' and to recognise their competence as collaborators. However, as is discussed later, this aspect of the HAZ initiative did not develop or sustain the profile which some hoped it would have and the emphasis on developing trusting relationships between organisations was greater than with communities.

Collaborative 'fit'

An important factor informing an individual's preparedness to engage with collaboration and to invest in developing collaborative capacity is the extent to which they understand collaboration as key to their career and working environment (Hudson et al. 1999). Many of the respondents interviewed were self-acknowledged enthusiasts for collaboration, people who had been waiting for the opportunity to work across the boundaries of sector and organisation. For them the experience of HAZ had enhanced their own capacity and helped to ensure that they were at the forefront of new developments at strategic, operational and/or community levels. However, for others who did not consider themselves advocates of collaboration pre-HAZ the issue of collaboration and its 'fit' with the current and future environment was a different proposition, one which it was not possible to explore fully in the HAZ evaluation and would benefit from further study.

The findings here seem to support Huxham's (1996) contention that collaborative action arises from a combination of selfish and selfless motivations amongst individuals. Those individuals who were most positive about the HAZ and their contribution to it were those for whom HAZ had provided an important opportunity to shine in career terms as well as offering a framework for action based on principles which they shared. The most obvious examples of those who experienced 'collaborative fit' were those high-profile leaders who moved onto more senior posts. However, there were other individuals in projects, at meso and strategic level who also experienced 'collaborative fit' with HAZ and were able to take up other opportunities as a result.

At the same time the fracture in the HAZ experience caused by the changes to policy priorities midway through the programme did interrupt this process and may have confirmed amongst sceptics their view of the transience of government's commitment to a radical programme such as HAZ. This acted to limit the ambition of individuals in HAZ and potentially undermined the developing collaborative capacity at local level. In some circumstances it also hastened the departure of HAZ 'stars' to other more secure positions in the public policy system.

Organisational capacity

Collaborative culture

The contribution of individuals to collaboration is insufficient if it is not supported by a wider commitment of partner organisations to developing new approaches. Sullivan and Skelcher (2002, p. 105) argue that collaboration requires 'host organisations to resource and support the development of a collaborative culture through the decentralisation of decision making and access to necessary infrastructure'. According to Newman (1996) organisations with 'collaborative cultures' are both 'adaptive and responsive'. This means that their orientation is outward to users and other organisations and their decision making is devolved to help facilitate a responsive mode within the organisation. The dangers inherent in such cultures are that such internal flexibility may result in an overall loss of control and that a strong external orientation could lead to fragmentation and a diluted sense of coherence. However, Newman argues that these limitations can be overcome if the organisation makes a significant investment in learning to improve its capacity and sustain itself.

In the HAZ context it became evident that it was necessary to develop a collaborative culture not only within the individual organisations that comprised the HAZ partnership, but also within the HAZ organisation itself (where this constituted a separate entity).

Collaborative culture as described by Newman was in evidence to different degrees in the partner organisations of the case study HAZs. In some cases, the evidence of collaborative culture was present in the language people used to talk about activities and programmes, regularly using 'we' to describe local action as opposed to emphasising the role of 'my organisation'. In Bradford considerable work had already been done in the district to develop an 'adaptive and responsive' culture through the restructuring of the council as part of its 'Community Government' programme of the mid-1990s. Under this programme the council adopted an area focus to its organisation, introducing Area Panels (made up of elected councillors) and area co-ordinators whose job it was to begin to 'join-up' council and other activity and to involve local people in decision making. While this programme had been effective in developing mechanisms for linking communities, other organisations and the council together at local level, its impact on the whole council culture was varied with the area co-ordination teams often seen as another department of the council. Part of the reason for this was the relatively limited amount of devolved decision making that accompanied the area programme. Decision making largely remained within central council committees and departments, necessarily limiting what was possible on the ground.

The other key aspect of a collaborative culture, the orientation towards users, was also variable among key partners. Health service organisations were generally considered to be less effective here than others including local government, and in its turn local government was frequently criticised for its failures and limitations. What was evident in a number of the case study HAZs was a desire to develop a more coherent and shared approach to community involvement/development. There were deliberate efforts to do this, for example in LSL, a key part of the HAZ strategy was to employ local community development workers to help provide a more coherent approach. However, while this greater coherence was being developed the activities of HAZ bore the hallmarks of the fragmentary and often partial approaches to community and user involvement that were a feature of many partner organisations resulting in frequently inconsistent and often non-strategic interventions – particularly in relation to Black and minority ethnic communities.

A considerable challenge to the collaborative cultures of partner organisations came with the 'modernisation' programmes launched for the NHS and local government (DETR 1998; DH 2000c; Sullivan and Skelcher 2002). In both cases (although probably more in the former than the latter), the ensuing reorganisations led to a move away from an external orientation and a greater preoccupation with internal concerns. The consequences of this were felt particularly in Bradford and Sandwell where reorganisation also meant a loss of coterminous boundaries.

In some contexts the HAZ itself was perceived as a separate entity. This could be either a self-perception amongst those appointed to work for the HAZ, or a perception of other stakeholders who experienced HAZ as one of many partners involved in supporting a particular project or initiative. There is evidence of this from all the case studies. For some the importance of understanding HAZ as a separate entity lay with its role as a change agent within the local health economy. Its potential capacity to influence change was considered significant although there were very often only a small number of people who could be considered to constitute the HAZ team.

One of the consequences of considering the HAZ to be a separate entity was that its existence could inspire envy amongst those who were committed to HAZ goals but were not HAZ team members and did not share in the perceived 'luxury' of being part of the HAZ team. This association was derived from the fact that some respondents saw the HAZ as offering key individuals the opportunity to spend time reflecting and developing ideas with other stakeholders and to test those ideas out in practice using HAZ funding. From their lofty vantage points HAZ people would then parachute into the 'real world' with their views on 'good practice' without taking account of the circumstances of mainstream providers, nor finding out what was already happening on the ground.

Learning

A collaborative culture is also a learning culture (Newman 1996). A commitment to learning was maintained by all the case study HAZs but its manifestation was frequently difficult to discern. Amongst individual respondents HAZ was frequently referred to as providing a 'breathing space' and an opportunity to learn. However, it was more difficult to find evidence of systematised approaches that would help sustain learning over time and across the HAZ. For example in Northumberland HAZ one respondent suggested that some of the missed opportunities to better co-ordinate activities within HAZ programmes could have been identified if there had been a more deliberate focus on learning in the HAZ. All of the case studies sought to use local evaluation in different ways and to different degrees to support local learning; in Bradford, for example, the local evaluation was a major investment for the HAZ over its lifetime; in Sandwell local evaluation focused on using multimedia methods to record the local experiences of the HAZ in 'Sandwell Stories' – an innovative but not entirely successful approach to evaluation. However, local evaluations were sometimes criticised by HAZ partners for not providing the right kind of learning support – this may have been a function of the changing HAZ context which meant that evaluation goals set at the beginning of HAZ may have been superseded by other objectives in the minds of the HAZ partners.

Whatever the reason, learning was often cited in HAZs as coming from different sources, the learning networks proposed by LSL, the HAZ-wide celebration events held in Bradford, and bespoke training programmes such as the leadership programme run in Northumberland.

For others, however, the opportunity to learn was not primarily through formal learning opportunities such as participation in training programmes or via evaluation feedback. Instead it came through the experience of participating in HAZ, of developing collaborations, working with users and designing and managing projects and programmes. Learning was passed on and carried into new environments as individuals changed jobs and moved on in their careers using their experiences to act as agents of change in new environments.

Organisational leadership

The development of a collaborative organisational culture requires sustained and targeted support. This highlights the importance of leadership in building the capacity of the organisation to act in collaboration and securing organisational commitment to this as a way of working. Organisational leadership then refers to the capacity of organisations to go beyond individual leaders to establish the organisation as a collaborative and innovative agent in its particular context. What is also important here is that different players are acknowledged as having an important role to play regardless of their size and status but rather based on their specific contribution.

In several case study areas the local health authorities were identified as important organisational leads in innovation and collaboration for health. The health authority/local authority relationship was also cited as key to promoting the health agenda more widely. Consequently the loss of these organizational leaders following health service reorganisation, which abolished health authorities and established multiple Primary Care Trusts in these areas, was considered potentially damaging. In some areas new mechanisms were established to try to recreate the strategic capacity held by the health authority. Elsewhere this strategic capacity was to be vested in an entirely new organisation. For example in Northumberland the new Care Trust was identified by many respondents as the strategic mechanism for promoting public health in the county.

Occasionally the capacity of organisations to lead was not matched by their capacity to embed innovations into the mainstream. For example in Sandwell the development of a whole district strategic framework for community involvement proved difficult to embed within partner organisations despite its endorsement by senior partners. This was in part because participants perceived that a communication gap had grown up between the senior partners and the front-line organisations which resulted in stakeholders questioning the depth of ownership of the strategy.

Occasionally the HAZ itself was considered a lead organisation. In MaST the development of this leadership capacity was driven partly by adversity and criticism and the need to present a united public face to defend the HAZ and protect projects and workers. Elsewhere, in LSL those not in the HAZ organisation considered that a core leadership function for the HAZ was the identification of key people in the local environment who might be important to achieving the goals of the HAZ and being proactive in 'keeping them in the loop'.

Inter-organisational trust

Lack of trust is often cited as a limiting factor in collaborations (e.g. Huxham and Vangen 2000). In addition trust in and between organisations is more difficult to achieve than trust between individuals. Cropper (1996) suggests that one way in which trust can be fostered in and between organisations is through what he terms 'principled conduct', modes of operating that provide the framework for collaborative action. Principled conduct will not substitute for the building of trust through experience but it can initiate exchanges between partners which in turn he believes can help to promote 'a sense of inclusion, of predictability or dependability, and of unequivocality in relationships' (Cropper 1996, p. 96). Cropper identified two elements to principled conduct – 'fair dealings' in relation to how the potential benefits of collaboration will be distributed and 'fairness in procedure', including the development of shared codes of conduct that organisation agree to abide by in their collaborative relationships.

The way in which collaborative benefits are distributed and the timing of those benefits are important issues in fostering trust, particularly across sectors. Sullivan and Skelcher (2002) argue that experience of funded area-based initiatives has shown that the less powerful partners frequently perceive inequity in the way in which collaborative benefits are divided up and the length of time community and voluntary sector bodies have to wait for their rewards compared to statutory partners. While not articulated in force across all of the case study HAZs, certain community and voluntary sector respondents reiterated this argument in relation to the operation of the HAZ with particular reference to the way in which decisions about resources were taken.

In relation to 'fairness in procedure' case study HAZs found the formalisation of codes or 'ground rules' for collaboration helpful and important. Unsurprisingly formal codes of conduct were developed early on in artificial or complex HAZs where there had been little prior collaboration. Formal agreements were said to help 'prevent misunderstandings' and to ensure that meetings did not 'get out of hand'. However, formalised arrangements were also evident amongst partners who had worked together previously and considered themselves adept at collaboration; here they provided a reminder of the shared basis for action that guided the collaboration. In some HAZs the development of 'principled conduct' was referred to primarily at the strategic level. However, in others 'ground rules' were considered vitally important in exchanges at all levels.

While formalised processes and practices were generally cited as helpful they could also be constraining. For example in Northumberland early formalised practices gave way to informal relationships and exchanges as trust between partners developed. For some respondents informal relationships were preferable because they permitted innovation and dynamic exchange more readily than formal arrangements.

Where the HAZ was considered a separate organisational entity its preparedness to take risks in innovation on behalf of the partners was one way in which it could build trust within the partnership (by demonstrating competence in action). One example of this was the work undertaken by LSL HAZ to develop and pilot 'developmental commissioning' a new approach to commissioning services that aimed to take better account of smaller, less powerful voluntary organisations. However, not all partner organisations were convinced of the value of this and this is one example of the problems of developing trust across a wide range of partners with different interests.

While these different approaches did succeed in building and sustaining trust between some partners, there remained scepticism particularly amongst voluntary sector partners about the depth of the partnership across sectors. Notwithstanding the development of agreed frameworks for collaboration and the management of the HAZ some voluntary sector respondents questioned whether all partners did play by the same rules. Examples were given of funding being allocated to 'big players' apparently outside the formal frameworks and justified on the basis of other rules and relationships that were external to HAZ and went beyond what could be captured in formal protocols.

Organisations and the 'logic of collaboration'

In the same way that individuals made decisions about the 'fit' between their personal aspirations and the collaborative environment the HAZ experience suggests that organisations too made decisions about their participation in HAZ based upon their judgements about the 'fit' between their organisation and the environment of HAZ. This can be described as the 'logic of collaboration' and it affects not only whether organisations will participate but also the nature of that participation and the construction of the consequent collaborative arrangements. It was the differing logics of collaboration in what may be termed complex and simple HAZs that contributed to the construction of HAZ as a separate entity in the former and as a collaborative process in the latter.

Logics of collaboration are not static but change in response to experience. So the initial emphasis in MaST on how to make collaboration work in an artificial environment gave way to a closer examination of why collaboration was important to achieve HAZ goals and what this might imply about appropriate collaborative relationships. One implication was the determination that in MaST it was necessary to work beyond administrative boundaries if necessary change was to be made. Elsewhere, LSL HAZ, another complex and to some extent artificial HAZ configuration, determined that entirely the opposite strategy was needed if change was to take root, that is it had to focus on the respective administrative units rather than the HAZ entity to achieve change.

So far this chapter has focused on exploring the rationales that underpinned HAZ strategies to generate collaboration and how they manifested themselves in those strategies. It has also examined the key components of collaborative capacity and their incidence in HAZ. In the next section of the chapter the evaluation data will be used to explore the impact of all this investment by examining the contribution made by the collaborative capacity generated in the HAZ initiative to the achievement of key HAZ goals.

Collaborative capacity and HAZ goals

This section addresses the four key questions that guided the 'building capacity for collaboration' element of HAZ evaluation. The first pair of questions concern the direct achievement of HAZ objectives:

- What contribution do cross-sectoral partnerships make to achieving HAZ objectives?
- What contribution does community involvement make to achieving HAZ objectives?

The second pair of questions relate to the interaction of HAZ with the new environment in which policies are designed and decisions are taken:

- In an environment where traditional tools of governance are being augmented or replaced by new instruments such as partnerships and networks (Sullivan and Skelcher 2002), what contribution has HAZ made to the development of cross-sectoral partnerships?
- In an environment in which citizens are urged to take responsibility for their own and others' welfare (Barnes and Prior 2000), can HAZs create the conditions in which community involvement meets the objectives of community participants as well as those of statutory agencies?

In responding to these questions it is important to reflect on the fact that 'HAZ' meant different things at different times in different places. Consequently it is hard to make conclusive statements about 'HAZ' generally. What must be understood is the way in which HAZ contributed to the dynamic change processes going on in each area of which HAZ was a part.

The contribution of partnerships and community involvement to achieving HAZ objectives

HAZ cannot be understood as anything other than a partnership-based programme. To that extent – in spite of conflicts evident at different points and the unequal experience of partnership amongst some groups and organisations – whatever was achieved was achieved through collaboration across organizational and sectoral boundaries. This can be illustrated in a number of ways.

HAZ supported the development of new models of service provision, to 'established' groups of service users. Examples here include the 'Repairs on Prescription' initiative in Sandwell which provided families of children with asthma with home insulation and central heating, and Performance Express – a project supported by Bradford HAZ which sought to build confidence and better health amongst users of mental health services.

HAZ also initiated the development of new models of service provision to groups who were previously poorly served or not identified as a priority for intervention in the context of health and health services initiatives. Examples here are Let's Get Serious in MaST – a project working with young men at risk of exclusion and becoming involved in criminal activity, and the Lambeth Play Strategy where LSL HAZ funded participative research with children to inform this strategy.

HAZ was also responsible in some areas for the development of closer links between health and community regeneration activity. The links made between the HAZ and Area Co-ordination schemes in Bradford; the focus in MaST on work in localities linked with SRB, Sure Start and NDC; and

HAZ funding of borough community development co-coordinators in LSL, illustrate the extent to which partnership supported by HAZ contributed to including a health dimension into community regeneration.

HAZ also acted to influence mainstream health organisations to work in more collaborative ways reflecting the ambitions contained in the HAZ strategies to build collaborative capacity. Bradford's strategy of supporting PCGs/PCTs through community involvement workers and funding work intended to promote HAZ principles is a good example of this. The development of the Care Trust in Northumberland was cited as the key legacy of HAZ partnership working.

Finally HAZ played a role in breaking down professional boundaries. Both the Sandwell Repairs on Prescription initiative and the teenage pregnancy initiative in MaST were illustrative of ways in which it was possible to support collaboration across professional boundaries and to limit the impact of professional defensiveness.

In many of these examples community engagement was also a key feature of the new ways of working that were being developed and which were starting to contribute to improved health amongst those engaged in these initiatives. There are other ways in which community involvement was instrumental in helping to deliver HAZ objectives. The experiential knowledge of community members made an important contribution to designing projects and developing strategies in many instances. For example, community led research in Northumberland was used as a means of increasing understanding of community needs; the 'Push Up' project in LSL recruited young people to seek the opinions of other young people on sexual health issues; and participatory appraisal and other methods of accessing community knowledge were frequently used in MaST development sites.

Objectives relating to the development of more participative forms of decision making and accountability were also facilitated through community involvement. This is discussed below.

The development of cross-sectoral partnerships as a mode of governance

Locating the particular contribution of HAZ to the development of understanding about the potential and limits of cross-sectoral partnerships as instruments for governing is complicated by the fact that HAZ partnerships shared space with many other partnership initiatives, their interactions informing their own development as well as their constituent partners' understanding of collaboration. In such an environment it would be inappropriate often to suggest that a single partnership – the HAZ – was 'leading' partnership activity. However, the HAZ was frequently identified as facilitating the inclusion of the NHS within partnership initiatives such as

NDC, SRB and Sure Start which otherwise might have been more difficult. In addition to working alongside and with other ABIs, HAZ also had to find ways of working with mainstream initiatives which sought to develop governance mechanisms which would support collaboration: in the context of HImPs, PCTs and towards the end of the period LSPs. In some cases the contribution of HAZ was important to the way in which these new mechanisms developed, for example in Bradford the HAZ encouraged PCTs to develop their collaborative capacity to work with other organisations and ABIs, and in MaST the experience of HAZ provided an opportunity to consider the circumstances under which partnerships across administrative boundaries would have some utility.

The experience of the five case studies supports Sullivan and Skelcher's (2002) view that collaborative capacity needs to be present across a range of sites if it is to become embedded (see Box 5.1).

The experience of HAZ also highlighted an addition to this list – voluntary sector capacity. This required the collaboration to acknowledge the role of voluntary bodies as equal partners in achieving shared outcomes and to build the necessary infrastructure to support this. The particular experience of HAZ and the potential contribution this makes to the development of public policy partnerships is explored below.

The constitution of HAZ decision making processes varied, in part in relation to the pre-existence of other partnership bodies through which it made sense to work. Such structures also changed over the life of HAZ. What did not change was that there was always an accountable body alongside the HAZ partnership where resources and authority for the initiative were vested – in the first instance the health authority and latterly, in most cases, one or more PCTs. In MaST, uniquely, a local authority took over this role towards the end of the period. Part of the process of mainstreaming was

Box 5.1 Sites of collaborative capacity

- Strategic capacity to establish a vision and to institute appropriate partnership bodies.
- Governance capacity to establish an appropriate constitutional form and accountability arrangements for the collaboration.
- Operational capacity to develop and employ new mechanisms for delivering services collaboratively.
- Practice capacity to draw on and develop the skills and abilities of workers to embrace and further the collaborative agenda.
- Community capacity to support the involvement of communities and citizens in opportunities opened up by HAZ.

Source: adapted from Sullivan and Skelcher (2002, p. 112)

to determine where authority for HAZ should lie. The problems caused by separate performance management and upward accountability mechanisms through NHS and local government channels were considered to place considerable constraints on local initiatives in this context. In particular the experience of the HAZs suggests that they were unable to progress very far in the pursuit of joint outcome measures because of the continuing dominance of the functional domains. In addition, trying to combine performance management with operational management, supporting organisational development and facilitating learning, proved very difficult for HAZs.

Different aspects of collaborative capacity were present at different times over the life of the HAZ. At strategic level there is little evidence that HAZ made a major contribution to solving the challenges of partnership governance (see Sullivan and Skelcher 2002, ch. 8). In part this was because the constitutional basis of HAZs (as 'unincorporated associations') offered relatively little freedom to develop new governance arrangements. While the experience of HAZ suggests that collaboration is essential to developing new ways of delivering services which will more effectively meet the needs of communities and service users, it also presents a number of challenges in terms of good governance including accountability for performance and accountability to the public.

HAZ was perhaps more successful in demonstrating the potential contribution of new governance mechanisms and forms of accountability beyond the strategic (the 'partnership board'). The experience of HAZ suggests that cross-sectoral partnership is easier to establish within localities than across broader geographical areas. It is also here that community involvement in governance processes was evident – at least in some areas. For example, within the MaST development sites community members were involved in, for example, decisions about the allocation of grants for health improvement projects; chairing and membership of steering groups and scrutinising the business case for a new health facility. In Bradford community members were involved in the groups developing healthy living networks and HAZ links with the area co-ordination work facilitated a health dimension to deliberation within neighbourhoods forums.

Operationally the HAZ also made relatively little impact in furthering the application of collaborative mechanisms. While HAZs did make use of certain mechanisms such as contracts, joint appointments and secondments they did not take particular advantage of the opportunity to explore more demanding mechanisms, such as pooled budgets or integrated services, except where progress on these issues had been made prior to the advent of HAZ, as in Northumberland. Again this may be related to the constitutional basis of HAZ and/or the fact that the initial enthusiasm for requesting 'freedoms and flexibilities' from central government dried up following central government's limited response to these requests.

Experience of developing infrastructure support for voluntary agencies to increase their capacity to play a significant role in collaborative governance was mixed. The importance of this was recognised and addressed in different ways, but although voluntary sector respondents felt that the HAZ experience had legitimised their role in local governance beyond that of service delivery agents there is little evidence that voluntary sector groups felt that they became equal partners in the HAZ enterprise.

Finally in this section it is worth reflecting back on the conceptual categories for HAZ strategies that were introduced at the beginning of this chapter, to consider what can be gleaned from these in relation to supporting the future development of collaborative capacity.

Consolidation strategies

Consolidation strategies are likely to be sustainable as they build on established relationships and ways of working. However, the danger of such a strategy lies in the potential for inertia. For example, HAZ did not mark any fundamental change of direction in terms of the approach to ways of working across agency boundaries and with communities in Sandwell as pre-existing mechanisms and relationships 'became' the HAZ. Arguably this contributed to the hiatus caused when major structural reconfigurations within the NHS created new 'partners' who occupied significant roles in the health economy but who were outside the loop as far as HAZ was concerned. Consolidation strategies can also fail to get beyond 'the enthusiasts', resulting in the possible failure of the strategy to impact on the 'core business' of partners.

Mainstream strategies

Mainstream strategies hold the potential for whole systems change, but could mean those outside the system remained disempowered. The 'managerial' approach to HAZ in Northumberland could be considered an example of this. Here the development of the Care Trust was cited as the most significant legacy of HAZ partnership working, but whilst there were many examples of community involvement in the context of HAZ, mechanisms for community influence on policy and service development remained relatively poorly developed. This suggests that for some partners such as the voluntary and community sector, mainstream strategies need to be accompanied by investment in infrastructure support in order to secure their effective participation. This was arguably less obviously the case in Bradford where the mainstream strategy deliberately emphasised building community involvement into the operation of PCTs.

Emergent strategies

Emergent strategies have the benefit of enabling a responsive approach in an unfamiliar environment. In MaST this meant a preparedness to change direction quite significantly when it became evident that the initial approach was not yielding significant results. It also meant that some partners were prioritised over others and some opted in or out at different stages in the HAZ. The limits of such a strategy include the lack of preparedness of some organisations to participate in activity which may appear incoherent and ambiguous, and the possibility of exclusive relationships developing as a result of prioritisation.

Innovation strategies

Innovation strategies offer the potential for ground-breaking work, but with weak infrastructure development which may mean that 'old ways of doing things' remain unchallenged by and impervious to new ideas and creativity. There may also be a tension between the freedom required for innovation and the discipline imposed by centrally determined performance management systems. All HAZs faced the dilemma of ensuring that effective innovative projects were sustainable and none sought to pursue an innovation strategy as a means of managing change throughout their life. In LSL it became clear that the notion that learning from innovation was the way to influence mainstream change was far from straightforward.

The capacity of HAZ to meet the objectives of community participants

Even in those areas where examples were given of community members being involved in processes that shaped the development of HAZ, there was also an awareness of the limits to this, not least because formal rules constrained the extent to which accountability for health services and policy can be expressed downwards to local communities. Overall HAZ became more of a top-down initiative than initial hopes and aspirations might have suggested. Priorities were set centrally in a way that was not originally anticipated; the need to respond to changes in the structure of the NHS and other policy and governance initiatives meant that more energy was expended in negotiating the place of HAZ in the context of the statutory system than in establishing community objectives and priorities.

Locally, statutory partners were not always aware of the extent of community and user organisations in existence nor well linked into community and user organisations. There were differences between HAZs in the extent to which they considered it important to develop an overall strategy for community involvement. In Sandwell there was an attempt to do so, but little evidence that this had been effectively implemented. In Bradford where there was evidence of substantial community organisation and activity, the HAZ strategy was to support this through organisational development within health service bodies, rather than focus on further community development. This strategy appears to have had some success. In MaST the size and diversity of the area led to a decision not to try to impose any particular model or approach to community involvement. Different models such as a social entrepreneur's approach and the more community development approaches adopted within development sites created particular opportunities for those directly involved. But there was no attempt to promote these approaches across the entire zone.

Some HAZ practices were regarded as exclusionary. This was the case with the early approach to project commissioning in LSL that led to an explicit strategy to address this through the developmental commissioning approach. There was also evidence of failure to understand the importance of developing mechanisms to translate community issues into action and to ensure feedback to those who had been involved. This was evident in, for example, the 'No Limits' young people's support project in Northumberland where young people had seen no tangible results of their participation.

Nevertheless there are examples of opportunities for community members to influence directions and where initiatives were welcomed by and supported aspirations of community members. In Sandwell the AgeWell initiative created a group of older people who became involved in deliberations about a range of issues affecting the lives of older people. Users of mental health services who became involved in Performance Express sang and acted out their aspirations in their own words and music.

But overall there was little evidence that strategic directions were shaped by communities or service users. On reflection, HAZ cannot be so strongly characterised as a community led initiative as a partnership initiative.

Conclusion

HAZs were conceived with a clear presumption about the value of collaboration to the achievement of the policy goals. This chapter has provided some evidence about the potential and limits of collaboration as experienced by local HAZs; subsequent chapters will further this discussion with reference to 'whole systems change' and health inequalities. However, the chapter has focused primarily on the significance to successful collaborations of the generation of requisite collaborative capacity to achieve stated policy goals. Evidence from the experience of the HAZ case studies suggests that there is no single approach to the generation of this capacity, rather that a variety of approaches will develop informed largely by the prevailing local context which both enables and constrains subsequent strategies for action.

Context is also vitally important in determining the way and extent to which local collaborations are able to develop and harness the key components of collaborative capacity within individuals and partner organisations. How collaborative action goes beyond those who are advocates and enthusiasts to those rather more reluctant participants, and indeed how far it needs to do so, remain important questions for research and practice. The significance of building in learning to collaborative action is certainly not a new conclusion but one that is strongly reinforced by the HAZ experience particularly in a policy environment where change is a constant feature.

What was also evident from the experience of the HAZ case studies was that there was no clear linear development from strategy to action to impact in relation to the generation and application of collaborative capacity. This was partly because the strategies developed by HAZ were concerned primarily (and arguably rightly) with collaborative action – how collaboration would manifest itself – rather than collaborative capacity, which would require an assessment of need and an audit of supply. Consequently what resulted was an interaction between strategy and context, between programmes of action and the skills and capacities of those individuals and organisations that could realise these programmes. For the evaluation team this marked an important feature, the preference for building capacity *through* collaboration rather than building capacity prior to collaboration.

Finally, while the evaluation explored a variety of aspects of collaborative capacity, it was the governance of HAZ partnerships that presented some of the most intractable challenges. These were centred upon the development of an appropriate infrastructure for accountability and in particular balancing accountability upwards to the Department of Health with accountability into localities to service users, citizens and communities (Barnes et al. 2004b). These challenges identified in HAZ have subsequently emerged in other ABIs and collaborative initiatives and their resolution will be important if collaborations are to remain as key instruments of local governance.

Chapter 6

Local strategies for whole systems change

Mhairi Mackenzie, Louise Lawson, Jane Mackinnon and Fiona Meth

Introduction

The HAZ initiative was located within a national policy context that recognised the cross-cutting nature of social problems such as health inequalities. As earlier chapters have outlined, this perspective had led to the development of a range of complex, multi-organisational and area-based initiatives that were informed by a number of assumptions about the policy route to social regeneration (Powell et al. 2001b). These assumptions included the following:

- Social problems such as unemployment, poor housing and ill health are inextricably linked and require joined-up solutions both across government departments, and between local partners.
- Local communities have an integral role to play in identifying the problems that are most salient to them and the types of solutions that might be developed to address these.
- Local partnerships can agree an overall strategic approach that encompasses an agreement of joint goals around identified problems, the development of appropriate activities to address these and realistic targets by which progress can be measured.
- Such partnerships will become learning organisations that will feed both formal and informal learning directly into ongoing decision-making processes.
- Joined-up local strategy development and implementation requires to be supported by joined-up policy making at a national and regional level.

In an analysis of cross-cutting issues affecting local government, Stewart et al. (1999) discussed the ways in which these kinds of assumptions reflect a growing understanding that a 'top-down control and compliance model' (whereby a centrally designed policy is imposed upon service providers and local compliance monitored) is not appropriate to the targeting of social

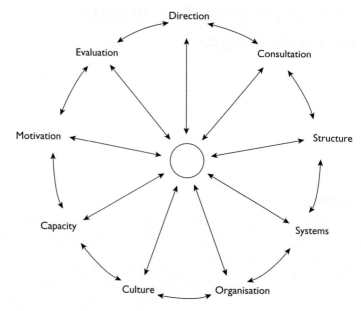

Figure 6.1 A model of whole systems change
Source: Stewart et al. (1999)

problems. Instead, the language of whole system approaches, derived primarily from the management and organisational behaviour literature (Bertalanffy 1952; Checkland 1981; Checkland and Scholes 1990), acknowledges the need to capture the kinds of complex relationships between central and local players and structures that need to be negotiated in identifying and addressing local and national problems. This has become a part of New Labour's policy rhetoric.

Recognising the centrality of complex organisational structures in delivering social change, the national HAZ evaluation (Judge et al. 1999), conceptualised the building of collaborative capacity (Chapter 5) and the development of whole systems change as necessary stepping stones en route to achieving measurable impact on health inequalities (Chapter 7). In this chapter we explore what is meant by whole systems change and discuss the progress made within a selected number of HAZs in realising change.

Conceptualising whole systems change

In their study of the effectiveness of partnerships established to bring about change within a range of policy fields, Stewart et al. (1999) utilised a whole systems model as a means of assessing strategic change (Figure 6.1).

This model has a number of strengths. First, it makes explicit those processes that have traditionally been taken for granted in the implementation of policy – for example, achieving a degree of clarity around an initiative's general strategic approach (direction). Within an initiative such as HAZ, the model would assume that local partnerships needed to *develop* a strategic approach to tackling health inequalities, and that such an approach could not simply have been presented to local players by central government.

Secondly, the model highlights the interrelatedness of various components in the change process. Thus, for HAZs, the nature of cultural shifts in health care organisations would have been partly dependent on the degree of consultation with partners and communities.

A third advantage of the model is that it recognises the importance of the interface between central and local change agents at each stage of the cycle. In other words, implementation success is not simply the responsibility of local providers. With HAZ, for example, communication between central and local bodies would not only have impacted on the extent to which a clear strategy was developed at the outset but also on the development of organisational structures through the establishment of Primary Care Trusts and Local Strategic Partnerships.

Finally, the model captures the evolving and potentially contested nature of most policy initiatives. The vision for the HAZ initiative, for example, may have differed not only between central and local stakeholders but also between and within HAZs (Barnes, M. et al. 2003b).

This model is useful for understanding the strategic approach and perceived progress of complex, multi-agency initiatives. For the purposes of understanding whole systems change within the HAZ initiative, however, the model has been amended in a number of ways. First, three stages in the process of bringing about systems change have been identified: strategy development and implementation, evaluation and learning, and mainstreaming. The three stages are, nonetheless, viewed as being closely interrelated, with a clear strategic direction impacting positively on the capacity to learn strategic lessons and on the likelihood of mainstreaming such lessons. Figure 6.2 illustrates the linkages between these stages and identifies some of the key components impinging on change.

Secondly, elements such as direction, structure, collaborative capacity and culture are considered to be salient at each of these stages. For example, whilst the importance of collaborative capacity is often emphasised at the strategic development stage, within this model it is assumed equally to underlie the processes of learning and mainstreaming. As we have emphasised in Chapter 5, collaborative capacity is built through working together, rather than in order to work together.

Thirdly, the adapted model offers the opportunity to view such elements as both drivers and inhibitors of progress at different stages of development within the one local context. So, collaborative capacity may have been

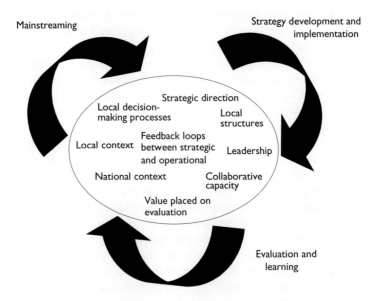

Mainstreaming

Strategy development and implementation

Strategic direction

Local decision-making processes

Local structures

Feedback loops between strategic and operational

Local context

Leadership

National context

Collaborative capacity

Value placed on evaluation

Evaluation and learning

Figure 6.2 A model of whole systems change within Health Action Zones

lacking in a particular HAZ at the outset resulting in poorly defined strategy. However, further down the road, an increased focus on building such capacity may have helped in developing a commitment to organisational learning.

Finally, these elements are conceptualised as being contextual factors, processes and/or outcomes within the one HAZ programme. That is, a strong culture of evaluation might be viewed as the context within which a joint health and local authority strategy for looked-after children is implemented, the process by which local decision-making becomes more 'evidence-based', and/or the outcome of a programme of capacity building among local project managers.

Utilising the model of whole systems change

One part of the national evaluation of HAZ focused on the process of whole systems change within eight case studies and addressed the following evaluation questions:

• What progress did the case studies make towards whole systems change?
• What were the factors that impacted on their capacity to develop a strong strategic approach?
• What were the barriers and drivers to embedding local learning and evaluation into their planning processes?

Table 6.1 HAZ configuration and population coverage at the start of the initiative

Organisational configuration	Wave	Population	Number of health authorities	Number of local authorities
Multiple-HA/Multiple-LA				
South Yorkshire Coalfields	1	770,000	3	3
Merseyside	2	1,400,000	4	5
Single HA/Multiple-LA (county and district)				
North Cumbria	1	320,000	1	5
Nottingham	2	640,500	1	6
Single HA/Multiple-LA (unitary)				
Camden and Islington	2	365,100	1	2
Coterminous HA and LA				
Leeds	2	727,000	1	1
Walsall	2	262,600	1	1
Sub-HA and unitary LA				
Luton	1	181,400	Part	1
Total	**8**		**12**	**24**

- What factors acted to inhibit or promote their ability to mainstream change?

A common thread running through the different aspects of the national evaluation is the importance of context as a determining factor in understanding change. The local and national context within which HAZs were operating was, therefore, a vital backdrop to these case study evaluation questions.

Chapter 4 describes the variation across individual HAZs in terms of size, organisational complexity, geography and population structure. Some of the most basic contextual factors as they relate to the whole systems change case studies are presented in Table 6.1, which highlights this diversity at the outset of the initiative.

In addition to a consideration of general strategic approaches within the whole systems change case studies, a more focused analysis of change in relation to children and young people (CYP) and coronary heart disease (CHD) was undertaken (Mackenzie et al. 2003). These topics were selected to represent the most commonly stated HAZ foci and activities based on documentary analysis conducted in 2000 (Bauld et al. 2001). Where appropriate, we use examples from these topics to illustrate the cycle of change within the case studies.

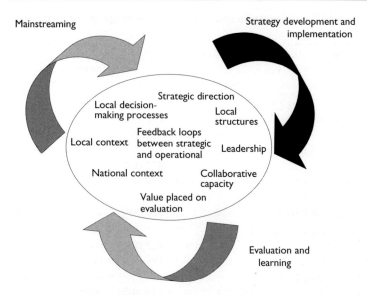

Mainstreaming

Strategy development and
implementation

Strategic direction

Local decision-
making processes

Local
structures

Feedback loops
Local context   between strategic
and operational

Leadership

National context

Collaborative
capacity

Value placed on
evaluation

Evaluation and
learning

Figure 6.3 A model of whole systems change within Health Action Zones –
strategy development and implementation

Strategy development and implementation

Here we consider the national and local contexts that impacted on strategic
development within the case studies and go on to discuss the approaches
used to inform strategy and its implementation. Figure 6.3 highlights the
key contextual factors that affected progress in the first stage of whole
system change.

The context: clarity of purpose at a national level

A central theme running through the literature in relation to strategic
development is the importance of clarity of purpose. Purpose is made up
not only of the stated aims of a centrally defined initiative but also of the
articulation of those aims as filtered through organisational understandings
at a local level (Stewart et al. 1999). There is no doubt that the *precise*
vision of central government in relation to HAZ was absent from the outset
and HAZs themselves had to respond to changing policy winds. In the real
world of policy implementation, local strategy makers anticipate such turbulence to a certain extent. It is fair to say, however, that an uncertain initial
purpose on the part of central government combined with policy changes
to the context in which all HAZ players were operating, made clarity of
purpose difficult at a local level.

The policy context for work around CYP illustrates this general point. Broadly speaking HAZ aspirations for the health of children and young people were congruent with government policy within other domains. So, for example, initiatives such as Sure Start, Quality Protects, Connexions and Sure Start Plus were based on the assumption that socio-economic deprivation in childhood and young adulthood creates long-term health and social disadvantage. From this point of view, HAZs were flowing with the policy tide.

This favourable policy context gave HAZs the reins in terms of tackling the wider determinants of health for this population group and provided the opportunity for joined-up approaches across policy domains within local areas.

On the other hand, the change in government focus in the early years of the initiative (Chapter 4) was perceived as a refocusing on a narrower NHS agenda and, for some HAZs, proved extremely disruptive in relation to the development of an overall strategic approach. Nottingham, for example, which had taken the decision locally to focus predominantly on children and young people, was forced to partially reinvent its approach.

Similarly, for those areas that chose to focus on CHD as a key area of activity, the national policy context was broadly supportive. The prevention of coronary heart disease is unambiguously a government priority. The White Paper *Saving Lives: Our Healthier Nation* (DH 1999d), for example, set a target of reducing the death rate from heart disease, stroke and related conditions by 40 per cent in those aged under 75 by 2010. *The NHS Plan* (DH 2000c) reinforced CHD as a clinical priority, focused on the preventative aspects of the disease and prioritised a reduction in health inequalities.

The more specific *National Service Framework for Coronary Heart Disease* (DH 2000b) set out the standards and services that should be available throughout England for the prevention, diagnosis and treatment of CHD. Its aim was to promote faster, fairer access to high-quality services and encompassed a reduction in CHD in the general population, prevention of CHD in high-risk groups and a focus on cardiac rehabilitation. However, as with work around CYP, the change in government direction in the early years of the HAZ initiative was perceived by many case studies as a return to a service and treatment agenda as opposed to a community and prevention focus.

The context: clarity of purpose at a local level

The responsibility to demonstrate a clear strategic approach does not lie solely with central government and not all individual case studies were able to demonstrate clarity at the outset of the initiative, nor had they put in place the systems through which such clarity might be achieved. Strategic development, therefore, was, in many cases, unfocused *prior* to changing

policy requirements. Indeed, in some cases, adapting to ministerial requirements and a perceived narrowing of the HAZ agenda after 2000 helped
some areas to find clarity of purpose at a local level.

It is important to bear in mind, however, that HAZs did not start with a
blank slate in relation to existing alliances, interventions and projects currently in play, or, the ways in which local health and social problems are
constructed. To a large degree these are the factors that constitute the
context within which strategies are conceived, shaped and evolved. This
context might consist of features such as an agreed need to develop city-
wide services for tackling inequalities for CYP, a series of small unrelated
but existing projects that might be gathered loosely under the banner of
heart health inequalities or a city-wide ethos of *Health For All* principles.

However, notwithstanding the policy turmoil that surrounded them,
some areas were able to maintain a focus on their identified purpose. Strong
partnerships and a real focus on *capacity building as a process* helped to
develop a sense of local HAZ ownership in some areas. This is not surpris-
ing since the need for shared values and vision in partnership working is
well documented in the field of health and social care (Rummery 1998;
Hudson et al. 1999; Rummery and Coleman 2003). (Strong partnerships
and good leadership within the whole systems change case studies are
difficult to disentangle; this is particularly true in areas where partner organisations were coming together for the first time as part of the HAZ
venture.)

Developing a local strategic focus is aided by a shared understanding of
the main health inequalities within a particular geographical area and the
prioritisation of activities to tackle these. By sustaining a focus on a small
number of workstreams of activity, some case studies were better able to
maintain a sense of purpose and to plan for mainstream change. South
Yorkshire Coalfields (SYC), for example, started with and maintained a
shared focus on CYP, CHD and disabilities, perhaps helped by a greater
homogeneity in its population than other areas.

Clarity of planning

As part of their performance management HAZs were required to use a
logical framework approach that summarised their key goal, activities,
milestones, indicators of success and targeted resources across their various
work programmes. The inherent rationale was that careful planning
around the likely outcomes of specified activities would help HAZs to
determine in the longer term whether they had made a difference and
would allow strategies to evolve as predicted activities and outcomes
changed. Whilst this was a problematic exercise in many ways, it provided
a window, however partial, into the detail with which strategies were both
planned and monitored.

As with many other initiatives of this type such as New Deal for Communities (Mackenzie et al. 2001a) and the Scottish Health Demonstration Projects (Blamey 2001; Mackenzie 2002), case study HAZs struggled with the task of planning activities and setting measurable early and intermediate measures of success. The following types of problem emerged:

- A lack of existing baselines hampered HAZs in setting the desired level of change that they wished to achieve – for example, in the nature of existing service provision or in levels of risk behaviours such as smoking in young people. Often the choice of target appeared to have been selected without the evidence of either routinely collected data or the identification of a problem through a needs assessment.
- Targets were frequently expressed with a lack of specificity that would make it impossible to determine if the HAZ had achieved its end. Some examples include 'reductions in cardiac-related disability'; 'reductions in pregnant women who smoke'.
- Selected targets were only a partial representation of the overall strategic purpose – for example, targets in relation to reducing a range of physical risk factors within a strategy that has an aim to develop better mental health services for children and families.
- Targets were felt to have been imposed on HAZs by central government and were not necessarily set at a locally realistic level because of a variety of contextual factors – for example, the likelihood of achieving 'a reduction of the number of deaths under 75 years of age from CHD by 40% by 2010' will be dependent on local demographics, existing service configuration and prioritisation of need.
- Activities and interventions were not conceptualised clearly enough to allow the degree of change to be predicted. This is the case both for focused work within both mainstream coronary and children's services and individual CHD and CYP projects.
- Process measures were not always plausibly linked to the types of outcomes predicted to emerge from them. For example, what was it about joint working specifically that would lead to improved health for looked-after-children?

There are, therefore, reservations about the degree to which HAZs were able to logically plan in a well-specified manner at the outset, but there are also reservations about the extent to which this was a reasonable expectation of them given the short deadlines for submitting plans. Later versions of strategic approaches as captured through performance management did not, however, suggest that these plans offered much more specificity in relation to their goals and activities. This suggests that initiatives require much more support in developing an integrated strategic approach (Killoran and Popay 2002).

Using the model of logical planning it would be reasonable to expect that the individual components of a strategy (be they processes, small projects at the margin of health care provision, major investments in existing service provision or large-scale refocusing on the wider health agenda) should add up to the aim of the overall strategy. Arguably, however, this is not a realistic expectation given the unknown nature of the relationships between possible elements (that is, the relationship may not be an additive one, rather it may be multiplicative or indeed activities may conflict and cancel each other out).

However, even with this qualification concerning the feasibility of highly detailed and prospectively specified strategic planning, there are many examples with the case study strategic programmes that simply did not add up. For example, one area that aimed to reduce inequality of access for CYP had a programme of activity that consisted of a number of projects dealing with issues such as breastfeeding, weaning, bereavement counselling and physical activity. All of these projects, however, targeted small population groups and were unlikely to reach the saturation required to have an overall population effect. A further example, taken from within one strand of a CYP work programme, was a well specified outcome in relation to reducing teenage pregnancy but where very limited resources had been identified to achieve this.

Given that evaluations of a range of different policy initiatives are reporting the difficulty that implementers experience in producing *logical plans* (that link the *central purpose* of the initiative to *feasible strategies* that will touch enough individuals to meet *measurable objectives*) then it is reasonable to ask whether this is a question of capacity and resource or whether it is inherently unrealistic to expect that plans can be developed in this way. Is the messy and changing world of policy implementation so contradictory to highly specified planning that it becomes counter-productive to place a huge emphasis on this level of planning (Barnes, M. et al. 2003a)? Of course, this is not to argue that planning, or a sense of direction, are not of paramount importance but that policymakers and evaluators require to be more realistic about the process of implementation and planning. Wilkinson and Appelbee (1999), for example, have argued that an overly programmatic approach to delivering change places an emphasis on top-down change processes that are to the detriment of 'lateral, cross-agency working' (p. 77).

Furthermore, if planning in HAZ was to have been taken seriously then local players needed *time* and *training* to engage partners and to focus on developing strategic priorities and solutions. Local planners also needed to have a sense that their plans were viewed within a national context as meaningful and coherent and that they would not be expected to overthrow these plans whenever a new national policy was launched. This required a *balance* between initiatives developing an overly rigid set of plans and central government viewing the HAZ initiative as the vehicle for taking forward all emerging policy relating to health and inequalities.

The usefulness of the performance monitoring data required by central government was contested. Some case studies found it useful as an internal monitoring framework, whilst others found that it clashed with their own local structures. Once again clarity of purpose is key. Those designing such information systems both locally and nationally required to be more explicit about *what data was for* and *how it would be used*. The collection of data *centrally* is only meaningful if it is seen to feed into decision-making or accountability processes in a transparent fashion. *Locally*, more thought needed to be given to how routine monitoring might more meaningfully be tied into the process of pulling together the overall HAZ picture.

Experiencing change across the system

Since strategic development is by no means only a paper exercise, it is important to consider the factors offered by the case studies in explaining perceptions of whole systems change in strategy development and implementation. A number of the case studies, for example, believed that a new way of working had been generated through the local HAZ. This was not viewed as a trivial change and it was acknowledged that the facilitation of the HAZ 'way of working' required to be resourced. Furthermore, it was felt to be greatly enhanced by strong leadership and by an explicit and strategic programme of activity that built these ways of working into the fabric of other partnership activities. Merseyside and SYC provide good examples of HAZs where strategic focus on changing ways of working was explicit from the outset; others such as Camden and Islington built this focus in as the HAZ progressed. Many representatives of partner organisations in such areas placed value on these changed methods of working.

Likewise, facilitation and leadership were required if the HAZ was to work at an operational as well as a strategic level. Without this, implementation gaps inevitably opened. Some areas invested in successful strategies to encourage projects to feel connected to the overall programme, and for those at a strategic level to be aware of *why* and *how* individual projects were contributing to the general strategic purpose. On the other hand, some operational managers displayed little sense of connection with the HAZ enterprise. The role of leadership within senior management is key in encouraging connectedness in both *vertical* and *horizontal* directions within an initiative such as HAZ. These kinds of feedback loops, as explored in Chapter 5, are identified as important ingredients in systems change (Chapman 2002) and are indicative of an adaptive style of leadership which emphasises the use of vertical authority to direct and support lateral connections within an organisational system (Wilkinson 1997; Pedler 1998).

An appreciation of the benefits of *commissioning* work non-competitively as opposed to instigating a *bidding process* for projects was considered to

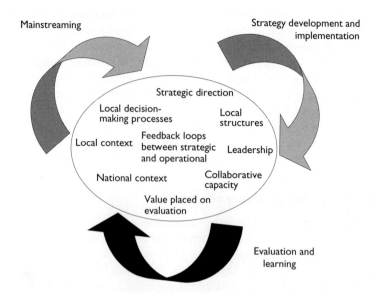

Strategic direction
Local decision-making processes
Local structures
Local context
Feedback loops between strategic and operational
Leadership
National context
Collaborative capacity
Value placed on evaluation

Mainstreaming

Strategy development and implementation

Evaluation and learning

Figure 6.4 A model of whole systems change within Health Action Zones – evaluation and learning

have been an important learning point across the case studies. In particular, its benefits are that it strengthened the linkages between individual pieces of work and the larger HAZ endeavour; it increased the likelihood that project learning would be viewed as important at a strategic level; and it lessened the likelihood of system overload when decisions of future funding were being made. It is important, however, that the commissioning process does not preclude the bottom-up identification of needs and solutions, an issue faced by LSL and discussed in Chapter 5.

Strategic development and its implementation represent a key phase in whole systems change. This phase is one where fruitful collaborations may be initiated, fostered, strengthened or damaged and which benefits from leadership and explicit resourcing. It provides the first test of whether holistic approaches to change were being pursued and whether these were supported by appropriate structures and systems.

Evaluation and learning

In the face of complexity, learning is central to systems change (Chapman 2002). In this section we consider the national and local *contexts* for developing HAZs as learning organisations, the *processes* and approaches taken to encourage learning and the types of learning *outcomes* (Figure 6.4 illustrates that the contextual factors impinging on strategic development also influenced evaluation and learning).

Here we utilise a definition of evaluation and learning that emphasises the substantial overlap between the two processes. Evaluation might be characterised as being a purposeful activity that aims to systematically assess the impact or operation of a project, process, practice or policy (Weiss 1998b). Learning, on the other hand, is a fuzzier, less formal process that both informs evaluation and is informed by it. It is an activity that is engaged in by individual practitioners and policy makers and collectively by organisations and initiatives. Like evaluation, the route by which learning becomes embedded in practice is neither straightforward nor inevitable. Decisions about policy and practice are made in a complex political, social and economic arena that does not necessarily privilege 'evidence' (Weiss 1998). Learning can be used within individual projects and by individuals without it ever being formally embedded within policy whilst evidence-based policy may not necessarily impact on individual practice.

The national context for learning and evaluation

At a formal level, evaluation of the HAZ enterprise was supported by the commissioning of research by the Department of Health. The evaluation team was charged with assessing the impact of the initiative in tackling health inequalities through modernisation of services and the building of collaborative capacity (Chapter 4). In addition, HAZs were established as learning organisations with the expectation that, at both a local and national level, systems would be established to encourage a culture of both learning from practice, and, of putting such learning back into practice. Again, this expectation, at a superficial level, fitted well with the push for evidence-based policy and practice espoused by the government both in terms of its modernisation of the mainstream agenda and, more specifically, in relation to the development of its various area-based initiatives (Davies et al. 2000a).

The way in which the learning approach was supported within the HAZ initiative included the funding of HAZNet, a web-based system that offered specific interest led networks, alerted subscribers to national and local policy and evaluation developments, and provided a route for dissemination between HAZs and their wider audience.

In addition, in order to engage frontline staff in learning and disseminating good practice, the National HAZ Fellowship Scheme was established. This scheme provided limited resources to allow a small number of individuals to develop a research project within their own area of practice. One example of this is the work undertaken in Luton to develop a means of encouraging age-appropriate weaning within the Asian community.

The national context not only offered some positive supports for the development of a learning culture but also raised barriers to effective learning. The frequently cited change in national focus, from a wider inequalities and bottom-up approach to a more top-down focus on national NHS priorities (Chapter 4), was perceived by the case studies as a constraint on innovation in practice and, therefore, of learning how to work differently. In addition, the performance management process was viewed by some as a barrier to effective learning because of its focus on outputs or outcomes. The degree to which the high-level statement documentation produced by HAZs for regional offices was (or indeed had the potential to be) useful in reaching national decisions about HAZ funding or focus is questioned by the case studies.

One element that characterises both the national and local context is the coexistence of a plethora of area-based initiatives. Stewart et al. (2002) discuss the problems that can result from different government departments and initiatives having different, and potentially conflicting, monitoring and reporting frameworks. HAZ and Sure Start, for example, operated very different monitoring frameworks.

Furthermore, the HAZ experience of an uncertain future and the speed of policy change both within and outside the NHS increased a general scepticism about the degree to which policy-making bodies were serious about learning from the overall initiative. This approach to policy making was not, of course, unique to the HAZ experience (Verma 1998; Nutley et al. 2003).

The local context for learning and evaluation

The local context within which the case study HAZs operated also provided both barriers and drivers to the development of effective learning systems. The degree of agreement about strategic direction locally and the methods through which this was reached affected the clarity of local evaluation strategies from the outset. In SYC, for example, the agreed prioritisation of young people, CHD and disability allowed a more focused development of an evaluation strategy in these areas. Where more amorphous strategy development occurred evaluation approaches were less likely to have been clearly focused.

The local context for evaluation and learning was also influenced by the extent to which information systems for monitoring changes in health outcomes and indicators were in place; the complexities of the organisational structures constituting the HAZ; and the existence of other area-based initiatives. The lack of adequate information systems made the establishment of baselines problematic and this had implications for both strategic development and evaluation of HAZ implementation and impact. Tackling this was more difficult in those HAZs where the geographical boundaries were not coterminous with those of their partner organisations. The ways in which the case studies negotiated and impacted on the local context for evaluation and learning are discussed below. It is important to reiterate that HAZs did not start with a blank slate and that they could be constrained or aided by the existing structures, processes and values around learning within their partner organisations.

The process: local approaches to evaluation and learning

The initial value placed on evaluation and learning within the case studies varied with some coming late to the view of evaluation as an integral part of bringing about whole system change. Most evaluation managers, for example, were not appointed at the beginning of the initiative and so strategies and systems for monitoring and evaluation were often being developed after the funding had been agreed for a range of projects, services and processes (for these projects, arguably, the question of evaluability was not high on the initial agenda).

The structures for directing and managing evaluation also differed markedly across areas, and, to an extent, mirrored the HAZ's view of the key purpose of evaluation. In North Cumbria, for example, evaluation at a strategic level was limited almost entirely to the collection of project management data and there was no dedicated evaluation manager for much of the HAZ's lifespan. In SYC, whilst there was no evaluation manager, a strategic level evaluation group was established in the early days of the programme and coordinated the evaluation activity of each of the HAZ's three work programme areas. A strategic approach to evaluation and planning was therefore built into the system. This was true also of Merseyside where a 'making it happen' workstream, that encompassed an evaluation strategy, ensured the prioritisation of learning processes within the development of wider strategy. In both of these cases, strong partnerships appeared to have been instrumental in sustaining an evaluation focus.

Nottingham, Merseyside, Camden and Islington, Leeds and Walsall employed an evaluation lead and these individuals had varying levels of responsibility for high-level programme monitoring. In some instances these individuals were supported by evaluation advisory groups. In Luton an academic researcher was employed who reported to an advisory group and whose primary role was to facilitate a small number of project evaluations.

There are three main components to the kinds of evaluation strategy that the case studies developed and these were pursued to differing extents. These are, as illustrated in Figure 6.5: building the capacity for learning at the individual project level; setting up formal monitoring systems across the HAZ; and developing capacity for whole systems learning.

For most (but not all) of the case studies, building the capacity of individual projects and members of frontline staff to self-evaluate was seen as fundamental to the success of the HAZ. Here self-evaluation was seen as beneficial for three distinct reasons. First, it would generate learning that would provide an impetus to mainstreaming good practice. Secondly, building local skills in evaluation was believed to lead to a sustained improvement

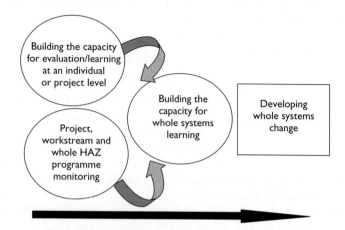

Figure 6.5 Components of strategy for evaluation and learning

in programme design and implementation within the local area. Thirdly, self-evaluation was viewed as a route to shared ownership of the overall HAZ programme. To this end evaluation toolkits were prepared and disseminated widely both locally and nationally (for example, by Nottingham, Merseyside and Leeds) and the training and mentoring of project workers, managers and workstream leads represented a key part of the role of some local evaluation managers.

Some of the case studies attempted to embed the HAZ principles of increasing community involvement and tackling inequalities within the process of building evaluation capacity at the project level. Some examples include the training of local people as interviewers for a survey of social capital in SYC and the funding of local community activists in Merseyside to undergo an evaluation training programme that incorporated work placements.

The national HAZ fellowship scheme is one good example of an approach to build learning capacity amongst frontline staff. This was augmented in some areas. Both Nottingham and Merseyside invested substantial evaluation resources in making local fellowship schemes work locally.

However, most of the case studies funded (either in whole or in part) a huge number of individual projects and so different sets of criteria were used to prioritise the projects for which support was given. In Merseyside, for example, these were around the resource intensiveness of a project, its perceived degree of innovation or its difficulty in meeting objectives. These were supplemented in Walsall with a criterion around the extent to which projects offered the opportunity to learn about complex change processes. In Leeds, on the other hand, a pragmatic decision was taken to support all those projects that received funding of over £10,000.

The rationale behind investing in project, workstream and overall HAZ programme monitoring is clear – monitoring is a means by which strategy implementation can be checked, problems identified, impact assessed and strategy refined. The case studies varied in whether they viewed monitoring as a central part of the evaluation and learning function. In Leeds, for example, the processes of evaluation and project monitoring remained sepa-rate whilst the evaluation leads in both Nottingham and Walsall had a role in pulling together HAZ monitoring data. Some HAZs, such as Luton, attempted to set up explicit systems to aggregate monitoring data from the project level to the overall programme level via the workstream level.

It is important to have a focus on, and make an impact with, both of these approaches to evaluation in order to build the capacity for whole system learning. The ways in which this tackled within the case studies included the organisation of learning events where those at a strategic level were brought face to face with frontline and project staff (for example, Luton, SYC and Merseyside) and the commissioning of programme-wide evaluations such as the focus on partnership processes in Leeds and Nottingham or the baseline social capital survey in SYC (jointly funded with Single Regeneration Budget funds). The development of evaluation fora where local evaluators from different initiatives shared learning about methodologies, toolkits and specific evaluations (Nottingham and Leeds are good examples of this) and the organisation of targeted discussions with policy makers in the new and emerging statutory organisations (Merseyside and Nottingham) provided further approaches to building the capacity of organisations and systems to learn.

The outcomes: types of emerging learning and evidence

At a project level a vast amount of data was generated, ranging from output monitoring, self-evaluation and reflective learning and externally funded evaluations. Those evaluation strategies that emphasised capacity building supported the approach of reflection and learning from problems in project implementation (Nottingham provided a useful example of this approach). The degree to which this was useful for individual projects and frontline staff was rarely looked at systematically and time will tell if evaluation aware-ness and skills were developed sufficiently to impact on future planning. Patton (1998) suggests, for example, that the process of being involved in evaluation helps people to clarify their goals and to think more evaluatively in the future. One example of an attempt to uncover the impact of a partic-ular evaluation approach is Nottingham's assessment of its local fellowship scheme – this study found the scheme to have been a useful way to enhance skills amongst frontline staff and a means through which future service delivery could be influenced, but, identified a range of local learning points if the scheme were to be extended.

For a number of projects, however, the types of monitoring data generated did not give a sense of whether project goals were being met (because the goals and indicators were vaguely expressed or because the indicators did not precisely relate to the goal). It is questioned whether this type of data constituted learning either for individual projects or for wider strategic programmes. Local capacity for evaluation at the project level was, therefore, weak in a number of cases.

At the overall workstream or HAZ-wide programme level, some HAZs made efforts to aggregate project data up to a planning level and invested in the development of joint information systems to monitor health outcomes and indicators. Luton and SYC, for example, used internal interim evaluations as a means of determining whether the overall strategic approach was having an impact. It is not always obvious, however, that learning emerging from the range of projects and processes evaluated added up to the goals of the overall strategy. (This issue is related to, but distinct from, the lack of connectedness between projects and overall strategies discussed earlier). A number of the case studies invested in systems-based events that attempted to take a holistic approach to learning across the HAZ. For proponents of a systems approach (Wilkinson and Appelbee 1999; Chapman 2002), this approach is important in emphasising the relations between activities at a horizontal and vertical level.

These types of events, whilst fostering a degree of connectedness within the system, did not always, in reality, relate back to planning and development. In many ways, therefore, the weakest component of evaluation strategy was the development of 'critical path approaches' (Beer et al. 1990) that linked activity at a project level into workstream objectives and then into wider HAZ goals.

Given their difficult starting place, it is important to acknowledge that many of the case studies developed learning systems that had the potential to make a difference to how evaluation and learning were perceived in the whole system cycle. Strong leadership and commitment to evaluation from the beginning of the HAZ initiative had meant that SYC and Merseyside were able to access and influence decision-making in the evolving health agenda using both informal and formal learning from the HAZ experience. In Luton and in Camden & Islington the evaluation approach that developed over time impacted on decisions about funding projects and practice around inequality. For example, Camden and Islington's whole systems learning events were perceived to have helped with the development of the PCT inequalities strategy. Without high-level commitment to learning, however, there is evidence of evaluation strategies that were struggling to make a difference, and where those who had dedicated time and energy to setting up systems for learning were fast becoming disillusioned with the rhetoric of evidence-based policy making.

Mainstreaming projects, processes and policy

A central aim for HAZs was the integration of services and approaches that had been developed through the initiative into mainstream activity. New Labour's adoption of special initiatives in pursuing 'joined-up' solutions to policy problems has resulted in the heightened focus on an additional implementation problem – that of how to 'mainstream' successful new approaches. Mainstreaming has become a buzzword in policy circles and requires be understood at a number of different levels. At its most basic, mainstreaming refers to the process of a project or service being taken on board by a core budget in a statutory organisation such as a PCT or local authority. Defined in this way, therefore, the mainstream is clearly distinct from time-bound, area-based or ad-hoc programmes that require new or distinct delivery agencies or ring-fenced funds; instead it is a longer term part of main service provision. However, in the context of area-based initiatives this definition has proved to be too simplistic. Because of the difficulties in securing such funding, mainstreaming is also taken to mean the continuation of funding by another organisation, with the implicit understanding that the longer a project continues, the more likely it is that it will become mainstreamed in the fullest sense of the term. Stewart and colleagues (2002) identified three levels at which mainstreaming can occur:

- *mainstreaming projects:* the securing of funding to continue particular activities
- *mainstreaming good practice or ways of working:* ensuring that a mainstream agency adapts and reproduces examples of good practice from an initiative or activity
- *mainstreaming policy:* when policy lessons from the work and experience of initiatives have a direct influence on the policy process.

The first of these clearly corresponds to the traditional definition of mainstreaming. The second level, mainstreaming good practice, implies that, whilst the initiative itself may cease, effective activities, partnerships or ways of working, would be identified, learned and adopted by mainstream organisations (for example, extending partnerships within the public sector to those who have been traditionally difficult to engage within the heath agenda). At the policy level, mainstreaming is best understood as transferring learning from a particular initiative or programme in a way that shapes future policy in the area. Thus it is important to distinguish between mainstreaming that occurs through the transfer of good practice from initiatives to local programme delivery on the one hand (for instance, using learning about consultation with young people across the HAZ to influence consultation strategies across wider service delivery), and mainstreaming that

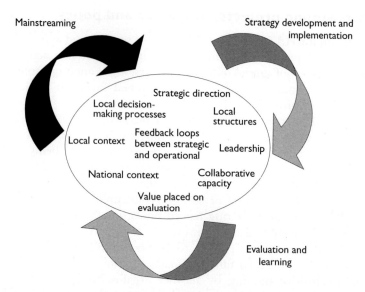

Mainstreaming

Strategy development and
implementation

Strategic direction

Local decision-
making processes

Local
structures

Local context

Feedback loops
between strategic
and operational

Leadership

National context

Collaborative
capacity

Value placed on
evaluation

Evaluation and
learning

Figure 6.6 A model of whole systems change within Health Action Zones –
mainstreaming projects, processes and policy

occurs from the transfer of lessons to national policy on the other. Whilst it
is at the policy level where mainstreaming is thought to be more influential,
and where lessons from HAZ can be best embedded, it is often at the
project level – securing continuing funding – that short-term effort has been
concentrated (Stewart et al. 2002).

Here we consider the context for mainstreaming health projects, practice
and policy and the extent to which case study HAZs made progress in this
stage of the cycle of whole systems change (Figure 6.6 illustrates the
salience of contextual factors impinging on mainstreaming progress).

The context for mainstreaming

The national context for HAZs, as outlined in Chapter 4, with its changing
goalposts and priorities and its pressure for 'early wins' operated against a
strategic approach to mainstreaming. At the same time HAZs were subject
to continued performance management requirements where they were
assessed in terms of their contribution to mainstream service delivery targets
such as reductions in waiting lists. Because of these pressures, Stewart et al.
(2002) suggest that local initiatives do not give the same priority to strategies for mainstreaming as they do to the preparation of delivery plans or to
implementation.

As time went on, the lack of clarity around the future for the HAZ initiative, structural changes within the NHS, and policy developments within

the wider regeneration agenda created a growing need to mainstream, and a plethora of new structures within which to negotiate such integration.

Mainstreaming: problems and progress

The *Shifting the Balance of Power* reforms indicated that HAZs were to be reabsorbed with mainstream health funding through primary care trusts (DH 2002b). Chapter 4 discusses the tensions inherent in this directive for the initiative and outlines the central importance of HAZ relations with their respective PCTs.

As with evaluation systems, those case studies that maintained a *focus on the mainstream* from the outset appear to have made most progress in impacting on developing structures such as PCTs and LSPs. Those that had a clearer sense of identity and purpose were also in a better position to embed their learning and ways of working within these bodies.

Success in mainstreaming projects was viewed by case study HAZs to have been particularly problematic where a bidding process rather than a non-competitive commissioning process was utilised for local funding. The constraints that led to 'projectitis' within HAZ meant that some areas struggled to know what should be mainstreamed and how criteria for decision-making should be set. In the same way as the HAZ initiative as a whole had been left awaiting funding decisions and, as a result, haemorrhaging key staff, so too had numerous local projects. Inevitably this led to damaging levels of cynicism. On the other hand, there were examples of projects which had been directly commissioned to address local needs and which perceived that HAZ resources, combined with an early opportunity to focus on health inequalities, meant that they had a greater likelihood of receiving mainstream funding.

There is some evidence that those HAZs that were closely integrated within existing structures were more likely to be successful in mainstreaming practice and policy locally. Examples include the city-wide children's strategy in Leeds that incorporated innovative models of care such as community-based paediatricians to reduce inequalities in access or Merseyside's CHD programme where improved service delivery was focused on targeting deprived populations and addressing specific local needs.

Mainstreaming at the policy level is believed to be not only the most influential route to change but also the most difficult to achieve (Stewart et al. 2002). Nevertheless, there are many examples where HAZs *contributed* in different ways to mainstreaming policy lessons and influenced a range of different agendas. Merseyside promoted local dissemination through a series of seminars targeted at commissioners from specific service areas as well as playing an advisory role at national level. Policy lessons from Leeds were mainstreamed by influencing decisions at local level and through dissemination of this learning at regional and national levels. Locally the knowledge from HAZ was applied to the Health Inequalities and Service Inequities Policy that was written to guide the work of the former health authority and, at the regional level, Leeds joined with other HAZs in the Humber Forum for Health and Regeneration to produce a good practice document entitled *Advancing Together for Health* (Humber Forum for Health and Regeneration 2000). The London and Luton HAZs pulled together their learning around project funding to propose a model of 'developmental commissioning' that would support innovation and increase the likelihood of mainstreaming (Vernon et al. 2002).

Whilst these examples illustrate the important learning from HAZ and the willingness to influence mainstream policies and wider agendas, there is less evidence about *how* policy lessons from HAZs were disseminated nationally and whether they influenced mainstream policies. Although the government remains keen to 'mainstream work on inequalities', there are still few mechanisms to enable this type of learning to feed upwards. Thus questions were raised by case studies about the commitment of national policy makers to take on board the lessons and learning from initiatives such as HAZ.

The timing of taking forward the learning from the HAZ initiative is particularly crucial. It is well recognised that the evidence base with respect to good practice from area-based initiatives often comes too late to influence further schemes and mainstream services (Stewart et al. 2002). There remained, however, a clear need to embed the achievements of HAZs in emerging structures and programmes, and efforts were made by individual HAZs and within central government to forge links with LSPs and PCTs. However, in the absence of sufficient investment and adequate connection, some LSPs were believed to be at risk of 'reinventing the wheel' particularly in relation to developing multi-agency partnerships and engaging communities.

The systems and supports required for mainstreaming projects, practice and policy are different. Once again this points to the need for strategic level and project staff to have been explicit about the mainstreaming *goal* of a piece of work from the outset. There were few examples of this within the case studies. Understanding the processes by which individual projects, processes and policies could be mainstreamed is not straightforward but needed to be understood by staff working at different levels with the HAZs. This again raises the need for *capacity building* for staff and organisations.

In summary, within the context of whole systems working, mainstreaming systems needs to be in place at the three levels of project, practice and policy if sustainable change is to occur. Whereas some areas were successful at mainstreaming specific projects, the overall approach of the HAZ was lacking in strategic direction and the procedures were not in place for taking forward the learning and policy lessons. Those case studies with a stronger strategy and more robust procedures were more likely to achieve greater success at mainstreaming at the three levels. The HAZs that adopted a 'mainstreaming strategy' at the outset were less likely to need to secure funding for specific projects as the focus was on changed ways of working. This suggests, therefore, that if a strategy is fully developed at the outset and procedures are in place for taking the learning forward then mainstreaming is part of the 'natural' process as opposed to a marginal add-on. Thus, locally, mainstreaming becomes part of the whole systems cycle and demonstrates the interrelatedness of the stages in the change model.

Conclusion

Three key requirements were necessary to achieve whole systems change and to translate the longer term aims of HAZ into practice. The first was an understanding of the cycle of change and its concomitant barriers/drivers at a national and local level. The second was a recognition of the part played by context (for example, in terms of local needs, organisational structures and capacity for collaboration) as the starting point for, and development of, any complex community initiative. Finally, there needed to be commitment to building evaluation and mainstreaming structures into the initial development of strategy.

The cycle of whole systems change with its contextual components is a useful model in understanding *how and why and where* the case studies were able to shift towards achieving success. An explicit recognition of context is fundamental in planning and learning about change. The national context, whilst supportive in some respects, created additional stressors on the whole system change cycle but, despite this, some HAZs created, and influenced the mainstreaming of, new ways of working. It remains to be seen whether these will impact on health inequalities in the longer term. The findings confirm Chapman's (2002) view of the need to view strategic change as complex and contingent rather than linear and wholly predictable:

> One way to visualise the difference between the mechanistic, linear approach to policy and the holistic, systemic approach is to compare the results of throwing a rock and a live bird. Mechanical linear models are excellent for understanding where the rock will end up, but useless for predicting the trajectory of a bird. To the degree that social and organisational systems, like the NHS, show adaptive behaviours they are better regarded as similar to live birds than lumps of rock.
>
> (Chapman 2002, p. 12)

Chapter 7

Tackling health inequalities

Michaela Benzeval

Introduction

HAZs were an important early symbol of the commitment of the New Labour government to tackling health inequalities. Moreover, the launch of the initiative was the first systematic attempt by central government to encourage local agencies to make reducing the health divide a core feature of their health strategies. Unfortunately, there was not a large evidence base for them to draw on, either in terms of specific interventions (Macintyre et al. 2001) or more general ways of working (Benzeval and Meth 2002a). HAZs, therefore, were expected to be trailblazers, leading the way in tackling health inequalities (DH 1998b).

HAZs were given two aims in relation to reducing health inequalities (Benzeval 2003a). First, they were meant to improve health outcomes and to reduce the health divide in their areas, and – since they were mainly located in disadvantaged areas – this was expected to reduce both local and national inequalities (DH 1998c). Secondly, they were expected to develop new ways of tackling local health inequalities (DH 1998b). To achieve this they had both to invest in innovative initiatives and ways of working and to establish effective ways of learning from them. They were expected both to mainstream lessons from their activities locally and to disseminate good practice more broadly within the health community.

The aim of this chapter is to explore HAZs' experience of tackling health inequalities. It draws on case studies carried out in three HAZs – East London and the City (Benzeval 2003b), North Staffordshire (Benzeval 2003c) and Sheffield (Benzeval 2003d). It begins by briefly summarising their approaches and achievements in relation to tackling health inequalities. It then considers the factors that affected their progress. Finally, it considers the implications of their experience for the policy process in relation to addressing health inequalities more generally.

HAZ strategies to tackle health inequalities

The goals HAZs set for themselves in relation to health inequalities varied considerably. For example, at one end of the spectrum was East London and the City HAZ, which was universally deprived, with high levels of average ill health and low levels of inequalities within its boundaries. It set itself goals and targets focused on reducing health inequalities by improving average health locally, aspiring to 'the next best similar area'. At the other end of the spectrum was Sheffield HAZ, with average levels of health close to the English mean, but with relatively high levels of inequalities within the city. Its goal was very much about reducing inequalities within the city, and focused on enabling all local wards to reach specified floor targets. North Staffordshire fitted in between these two approaches with its overall goal focusing on differences between the HAZ and the national average, while some of its targets also focused on improving health outcomes in the worst wards.

Despite the articulation of these outcome goals, there was a general belief across the HAZs that reducing inequalities in health outcomes in the medium term was not achievable for two main reasons. First, HAZ resources were not seen to be sufficient to make significant changes in the lives of their populations. Secondly, the timescale of the HAZ initiative was believed to be too short to achieve sufficient changes in the long-term causes of inequalities. Given this, over time most stakeholders came to see the HAZ's role as being to develop the local capacity to address health inequalities.

The role HAZs played in tackling health inequalities locally

In many ways, HAZs were an advanced microcosm of the general policy framework that New Labour introduced for all local health authorities to address health inequalities. For example, the requirement to make tackling health inequalities a priority; giving explicit responsibility to local agencies to do this and holding them to account for their actions; the emphasis on partnership working and community involvement; and, the recognition of the need to develop an evidence base about how to reduce inequalities, were all part of the wider framework for addressing health inequalities introduced during New Labour's first term in office (Benzeval and Meth 2002a). In addition, however, HAZs had three key extra mechanisms with which to tackle health inequalities:

- ring-fenced funding
- a dedicated policy space
- being a status symbol.

Drawing on all three of these mechanisms HAZs were, at some points in time in some places, able to act as catalysts or drivers for change in relation to particular needs within their local health economies. The ways in which the three HAZs, described in this chapter, made use of these mechanisms to enhance their local capacity to address health inequalities are highlighted below.

Ring-fenced funding

HAZ funding played a number of valuable roles in enhancing local capacity to tackle health inequalities.

Firstly, it enabled the local health economy to invest in services and issues that were not priorities for mainstream services. For example, HAZs funded activities beyond the traditional remit of the health services to address some of the determinants of health such as poor housing, low incomes and unemployment. Within the health service arena, they supported health promotion and prevention activities, community development and other social support initiatives. HAZ funding also enabled the local economy to target services at areas and vulnerable groups in ways that was not possible within mainstream resources. In doing this, HAZs created flexibility or 'elbow room' for local partners to focus on local priorities that were not the subject of central government targets. There was widespread belief among key stakeholders that the ability to invest additional resources in areas or groups with higher needs was crucial to any strategy to reduce health inequalities, but that this was not possible without additional ring-fenced financing.

Secondly, HAZs invested resources in publicising key local problems and different kinds of initiatives. They funded analyses of health inequalities problems, produced a wide range of different kinds of publications, newsletters and websites, and organized high-profile events and other public relations activities to generate media attention and public interest.

Thirdly, HAZ resources facilitated and enabled local innovation and experimentation. This involved supporting good ideas, people and organizations; placing an emphasis on the need for piloting and learning; and, allowing services to 'double run' experiments alongside current activities to test and refine them before trying to introduce wholesale change. Fourthly, in a range of ways the additional HAZ funding 'oiled the wheels' of local partnership activities, for example, by supporting mainstream posts and service developments; through the work of the HAZ team; and, in some cases, by bringing into the local economy a range of different consultants and facilitators.

However, against this positive perception, concern was expressed that the HAZ money had simply been used to 'plug a few gaps', particularly in relation to NHS priorities. HAZ resources were considered a 'drop in the ocean' in relation to local needs in terms of tackling health inequalities, and as such were seen as a distraction from the key ways in which the HAZ could contribute to local efforts to reduce health inequalities. Moreover, in one HAZ, senior managers in the PCTs and the LAs felt that the cost of the HAZ, in terms of their time, was far greater than the benefits that HAZ status had conferred locally.

A dedicated policy space

Across the HAZs, the initiative was felt to have created a policy 'space' particularly focused on health inequalities. While there was a general increase in policy attention nationally in relation to health inequalities (Benzeval and Meth 2002a), being a HAZ was felt to have added value by bringing a clearer and stronger focus and commitment to tackling them. For both agencies and individuals the HAZ legitimised activities concerned with reducing health inequalities, in ways that were not possible within the mainstream. It was described as an 'introductory agency' bringing together different individuals and groups across the broad spectrum of organisations that could have an impact on health. It created opportunities for people to network with like-minded colleagues to discuss new ways of working to tackle health inequalities as well as to work together on practical projects. It also created an intellectual space for individuals to think about health inequalities in ways that were not possible in their day jobs, to 'think bigger' and/or 'outside their usual boxes'. For individuals who interacted with the HAZ, it created valuable opportunities to develop their skills and experiences. For example, HAZs provided training in project management, planning and evaluation. They created opportunities for people to have new leadership roles within local partnerships and projects, and to try working in a range of different ways. (This supports findings in relation to some of the contributions HAZs made to developing collaborative capacity locally: see Chapter 5.)

Being a status symbol

The status of being a HAZ was seen as important recognition of the problems that the different areas faced. This helped to create a focus on health inequalities locally, which it was felt might not otherwise exist. In addition, the HAZ 'badge', at least in the early days of the initiative, was felt both at the strategic level and at the project level to be useful in levering additional resources into the area.

Bringing it together: HAZ as a driver for change

Drawing on the extra funding that they received, the policy space that they were able to create for health inequalities and the leverage that being a HAZ gave them, at some points in time in some places, HAZs were able to be 'drivers for change' in the local economy. In a general way, HAZs focused a 'spotlight on public health' issues locally. These were not particularly new issues, but local champions were able to use the HAZ as an important policy vehicle to push forward issues that they were already concerned with.

More specifically, HAZs combined the resources and space that they were given to act as catalysts for change in relation to a number of local processes and structures. In North Staffordshire, the HAZ developed a number of 'tools' – for example, logical planning frameworks and a partnership audit. The HAZ as a 'tool box' was a frequently cited mantra among stakeholders. In East London, the HAZ was a catalyst for change in strategic partnership arrangements locally. It facilitated a shift to locality partnerships, which had much greater local ownership than the East London wide structures. In Sheffield, initially at least, the HAZ was seen as an 'engine room of change', a 'research and development programme' to innovate, to evaluate and to learn about new ways to tackle health inequalities. The aspiration had been to extract learning about what works from 'illustrative projects' and 'industrial scale' this to mainstream services. All three HAZs saw an important part of their role as being to develop the evidence base about what works in reducing health inequalities. But for a range of reasons, in particular changes in central government policy, this experimental development role was difficult. Nevertheless, in Sheffield, in particular, the emphasis on evaluation and the support that the HAZ provided for this were believed by a range of stakeholders to have improved the capacity for learning locally.

The impact of the HAZs

The government and individual HAZs saw changes in ways of working locally – to better enable local areas to address health inequalities – as being an important goal for the initiative. In this respect the contribution that each HAZ made very much reflects the local context: the starting point for the HAZ in terms of the existing commitment to addressing health inequalities and understanding of how to do so; the extent to which integrated partnerships were already working together on health issues; and, the capacity of the changing set of actors and agencies to contribute to, and learn from, the HAZ experience. Nevertheless, there are some general ways in which the three HAZs developed local capacity for tackling health inequalities; albeit to differing degrees and from different starting points.

First, the activities and existence of HAZs in a particular location were felt to have made health inequalities a much more visible issue and hence pushed it up the local agenda. HAZs increased awareness of health inequalities locally and ways of addressing them. One particular aspect of this, which was praised by a number of stakeholders across the HAZs, was the way that HAZs had supported and hence raised the profile of particular, often hidden or neglected, issues and groups within the local policy arena.

Secondly, HAZs were felt to have promoted a greater understanding of the determinants of health and of the range of partners necessary to address health inequalities. The extent to which it was felt that a shared understanding of the social model of health had been achieved was related to the level of understanding that existed before the HAZ. Nevertheless, in all three HAZs, the understanding of the causes of health inequalities was felt to have broadened as a result of its activities. However, in one HAZ, where there was felt to be only a limited 'public health mindset' to begin with, many people acknowledged that considerable further work was required to 'win hearts and minds' in the local policy community.

Linked to this, HAZs had increased understanding not only of the need for partnership working to tackle health inequalities but also of the ways in which this could be done within the local context. The process of working together at different levels was felt to have promoted a better understanding of the different cultures and constraints that partners work within, enabling them to work together more effectively in the future.

The three HAZs also contributed to the ongoing development of underlying structures and processes in their localities. This included developing local capacity for running whole systems events, for logical planning and evaluation, for involving communities in decision-making, and for partnership working. (The ways in which other HAZs attempted to promote these ways of working are discussed in more detail in Chapters 5 and 6.) In areas where a significant infrastructure existed before the HAZ, it appeared to make less of a contribution than those where the existing structures, capabilities and processes were more limited.

For individuals, engagement with HAZ activities was felt to have improved informal networks and developed significant personal connections with other people sympathetic to reducing health inequalities. A range of stakeholders commented on the significant personal development opportunities created for them by being connected to the HAZ.

Finally, at the local level, HAZs were felt to have made significant changes to the delivery of some mainstream services in the area in ways that should improve the quality of and access to services for local communities. In some, but not all, cases such developments were particularly focused on designing specific services that would better meet the needs of disadvantaged areas or groups, so that such improvements would reduce inequalities in access to care.

Inhibiting and facilitating factors

The importance of different factors in the local context influencing policy formulation and implementation has been identified in studies across a range of fields and settings (e.g. Pettigrew et al. 1992; Evans and Killoran 2000; Abbott et al. 2001; Mays et al. 2001; Milligan 2001). Such contexts change over time (Pettigrew et al. 1992) and the relationship between context and policy can be two-way (Dahler-Larsen 2001), that is HAZs may have affected their local context in ways that hindered or facilitated the future implementation of their own activities (Benzeval 2003a). Four sets of factors appeared to affect the progress of these three HAZs in relation to tackling health inequalities. These were:

- the nature of the problem
- organisational configurations and histories
- the public sector labour market
- the role of key personalities as champions and blockers.

In addition, as discussed in previous chapters, changes in the national policy context also influenced the impact of the HAZs locally.

The nature of the problem

A number of issues about the particular manifestation of health inequalities locally, as well as specific underlying causes, posed challenges for the HAZs.

Within the HAZs' territories, a range of different problems existed cheek by jowl – affluence and poverty, urban and rural landscapes. These different kinds of areas had different needs and required different policy solutions. However, central policy dictates often prioritised one over another (e.g. urban issues over rural ones) contrary to local perceptions of problems. The blanket approach of many ABIs more generally has been criticised for ignoring the different manifestations of problems in different places (Martin 2001). A related issue was that the available data and techniques to identify places or groups experiencing disadvantage were often rather blunt instruments. Often administrative units – such as LA areas or wards – were used to target resources at communities of disadvantage or interest. While in some cases these boundaries mapped together well, in others they were rather crude approximations, missing more of those in need than identifying them, again echoing similar debates about the merits of ABIs more generally (e.g. Powell et al. 2001a).

A second important aspect of the local contexts that influenced the HAZs' task, resulted from their differing social and economic histories, which in turn led to different kinds of health problems. In Sheffield and North Staffordshire the decline of local industries had left high numbers of unskilled workers without jobs; many with industrial-related diseases, for example, high rates of respiratory disease as a result of mining. In East London, the significant and ever-growing minority ethnic population presented local agencies with a range of challenges that were atypical nationally. Again, the national priorities set for HAZs sometimes made it difficult for the HAZ to give priority to local manifestations of key problems.

The causes of health inequalities in general are complex, but in some areas the interaction of a whole host of different social and economic problems meant the size of the task facing HAZs was immense. In such circumstances, local stakeholders found it difficult to prioritise; all problems needed attention. But this resulted in the HAZ spreading its resources rather thinly, perhaps reducing its potential impact over all.

Organisational configurations and histories

Each of the HAZs faced problems as a result of the changing configuration of the geographic boundaries of its partners and local historical relationships. Coterminosity, in particular, has been shown to be an important facilitating factor in joint working across a range of studies (e.g. Exworthy and Peckham 1998; Fulop et al. 1998; Stewart et al. 1999). Neither East London and the City nor North Staffordshire HAZs were felt to be 'natural communities'. There was a lack of history of joint working across the geographic areas covered by the HAZ, and relevant LAs could see little value for themselves in working with other geographically based organizations. A shared history has been shown as being important for building ownership of an initiative in a broader review of ABIs (DETR 2000a). The building capacity for collaboration component of the HAZ evaluation also found that partnerships were easier to establish within commonly defined localities than across administrative boundaries (Chapter 5).

In North Staffordshire, this problem was exacerbated by the involvement of both unitary and two-tier councils, and by the HAZ being focused on the urban areas only, meaning that it covered only parts of three of the four LAs involved in the HAZ. For these agencies the HAZ covered only a small part of their responsibilities, so it was difficult for them 'to bend' mainstream resources to address HAZ priorities or take on board lessons from the HAZ experience. It also created tensions within those agencies, when HAZ resources were being spent on an initiative in one part of their region, but they felt another area was at least as in need of such investments. In East London, while all of the constituent LAs were included within the HAZ, there was again a feeling that each LA had particular needs that were not shared across the HAZ. Historically competitive relationships between the LAs, as they had bid against each other for central government support, added to the reluctance of local councillors to see value in working with other LAs. Similar problems have been identified for other HAZs as a result of the histories of the territories that they covered (Painter with Clarence 2001).

The devolution of planning and commissioning health care to PCTs in East London resulted in coterminosity between the health service and LAs, and in North Staffordshire, the boundaries of the PCTs and LAs are nearly but not quite coterminous. In Sheffield, on the other hand, while the HAZ originally benefited from coterminous relations between its health and local unitary authority, the HA responsibilities were devolved to four PCTs, breaking up this much-valued coterminous partnership. Views were divided in the city about the extent to which this might lead to problems in partnership working (see Chapter 5 for further discussion of these issues).

All three areas covered by the HAZs had a history of partnership working, although tensions were apparent in each of these. There were the general cultural problems in collaborations between the health sector and local authorities (e.g. Hiscock and Pearson 1999), and in developing meaningful ways of engaging with users and communities (e.g. Cook 2002). Further tensions arose in two of the HAZs as a result of the Healthy Cities initiative already being established. In addition, the territories covered by the HAZs, especially East London and the City and Sheffield, were subject to a plethora of other area-based partnership initiatives, creating confusion and overloading local agencies (DETR 2000a).

An additional tension was created as a consequence of resources and accountability being channelled through the NHS, such that HAZs were often seen as an NHS entity rather than a true partnership endeavour. These perceptions were exacerbated when the change in HAZ priorities increased the amount of resources being spent on NHS issues.

All of these different issues meant that HAZs entered a crowded partnership arena in which tensions already existed among some of the key players. For some HAZs these tensions were initially exacerbated by, and also affected, their development and ownership. In one HAZ in particular, this made the partnership a rather difficult structure to be involved with. Nevertheless, some of the conflicts that were resolved there are believed to have improved the foundation for partnership working in the future. For the HAZ itself, however, this meant it struggled to be a key vehicle for tackling health inequalities locally, and, in particular, for initiating change in mainstream agencies because of a lack of ownership and trust within the partnership.

The public sector labour market

The public sector labour market faced by the three HAZs varied in important ways. In East London, there was a tight labour market with a high rate of staff turnover at all levels and a shortage of staff. All of the statutory agencies faced problems with both recruitment and retention. This had a number of different consequences for the HAZ. Firstly, at any one time staff vacancies meant that all other staff were stretched to or beyond capacity, making adding HAZ activities to their day job difficult. Secondly, the high turnover of staff created continuity and ownership problems, often despite the best endeavours and huge commitment of other individuals.

Thirdly, concern was raised about the consequences for organizational learning locally from the HAZ, when many key people involved had moved on to new jobs outside of the area. Evans and Killoran (2000) also found high staff turnover to be a disabling factor in local efforts to address health inequalities.

In contrast, the level of staff turnover in Sheffield and North Staffordshire was much lower, with key staff at all levels having worked within the area for long periods of time. In Sheffield there was concern that this made the health economy rather 'cliquey' and that for some key individuals the 'baggage' of past jobs and working relationships affected their new roles. The history, as well as the current role, of key actors has been identified as an important factor in the dynamics of local policy networks in other studies (Milligan 2001). In North Staffordshire some local agencies were felt to be rather inward looking and 'conservative' and, as a result, unwilling to embrace new ideas and change. For Sheffield, this meant some old tensions were played out around the HAZs' role, while in North Staffordshire it sometimes made it difficult for the HAZ to introduce new ideas and take mainstream agencies with them.

The role of key personalities as champions and blockers

Across the HAZs, the role of key individuals in enabling or inhibiting the development and achievements of the HAZ, and particular workstreams or initiatives within it, was highly significant. Many stakeholders felt that the HAZ had been used effectively by different champions to push forward the health inequalities agenda generally, or specific aspects of it with which they were already concerned. In some cases such people were good networkers, making connections and fostering relationships to support the partnership process (the importance of such reticulists and boundary spanners is discussed in Chapter 5). In other cases, they had the vision to see the opportunities the HAZ created and used them to open doors, get issues on agendas, lever resources into the system and bring about change. However, each of the three HAZs also had significant personalities who were seen as blockers, for example, by skewing HAZ priorities away from those shared by the broader partnership and by generally being unsupportive and not valuing the contribution of the other partners.

As in other studies the status of both champions and blockers (Stocking 1985; Stewart et al. 1999; Milligan 2001), and hence the power they had in local networks, was a significant factor in HAZ fortunes. The loss of key leaders, as occurred in all three HAZs, can have a detrimental effect on progress (Stocking 1985; Pettigrew et al. 1992; Mays et al. 2001). On the other hand, new opportunities were created for the HAZs as some of the individuals acting as blockers moved on.

Changes in the national policy context

As discussed in Chapter 4 changes in national policy relating to HAZs specifically, and more generally, had a significant effect on the local fortunes of the HAZs. Initially, there was enormous enthusiasm for the HAZ idea in general, and tackling health inequalities in particular, among many stakeholders. Local leaders used this to push key issues onto local agendas. However, in all three HAZs, the change in central priorities and the subsequent funding uncertainty, both of which made it appear that HAZs had fallen off the national agenda, had a detrimental effect on their local ownership and hence their ability to fulfil their goals. The three HAZs reshaped their programmes and plans to better match the government's revised priorities (Benzeval 2003a). There was a perception that this shifted them away from tackling issues around the root causes of ill health and inhibited their ability to innovate and to invest in evaluation, as well as reducing attention on local priorities in favour of central NHS ones. Nevertheless, local HAZ leaders used new national policy announcements, such the launch of the national inequalities targets or consultation document on inequalities, to lever health inequalities back up the local agenda. The ability of leaders to seize on key aspects of the changing context to push forward the agenda is an important factor in making progress locally (Pettigrew et al. 1992).

More broadly, the significant changes in HAZ partner agencies undermined the HAZs' ability to influence issues, as the general organizational turmoil drew attention away from HAZs and their change agendas. This disruption has been noted in a range of other studies of local efforts to promote health and reduce health inequalities (e.g. Hunter et al. 1998; Evans and Killoran 2000; Benzeval and Meth 2002a).

Issues for the policy process

The experience of HAZs in trying to develop local approaches to address health inequalities raises a number of issues for policy. Some of these are specific to the nature of the health inequalities problem and others reflect broader issues associated with tackling complex social problems at the local level.

Understanding health inequalities: the problem, the causes and the solutions

Goals

HAZs' experience of health inequalities and their interpretation of the broad goal – 'to reduce health inequalities' – set by government varied considerably. Ambiguity in health inequalities goals has been noted at both the national level (Graham 2004) and the local level in England (Benzeval and Meth 2002a). Humpage and Fleras (2001) argue that such ambiguity at the national level, in New Zealand at least, has been helpful in creating broad coalitions in relation to health inequalities. Ambiguity in national policy can allow different interpretations at the local level relevant to local needs (Hill 1997). Both of these benefits were apparent in the HAZs' experiences. A broad range of stakeholders were attracted to the HAZs because of their commitment to address health inequalities, with many special interest groups seeing the HAZ as a way of pushing their concerns up the agenda. The ambiguity of the national goal for HAZs enabled each HAZ to develop its own inequalities goals relevant to the particular manifestation of causes and consequences locally. However, the breadth of possible interpretations of the national goal also contributed to some of the difficulties the HAZs experienced in agreeing their strategies.

The nature of the health inequalities problem, and understanding of it, had a significant effect on the coherence and ownership of the HAZ strategy, and hence the commitment to supporting it. For example, in Sheffield, there was a clear understanding of the goal of reducing inequalities within the city and hence the HAZ's strategy to invest most of its resources in the most disadvantaged areas had general support. As a result, significant areas of the city did not receive HAZ investment, which caused unhappiness among organizations representing such places. There was also concern that the initial approach used by the HAZ to identify such areas was rather crude, and hence this was subsequently refined. In East London, where there was consensus about the universal nature of the problem, there was concern that the subsequent general focus on improving average levels of health was ignoring more subtle variations in need within the area.

The HAZ experience, therefore, reflects that of other efforts to address complex social problems. For example, in a review of initiatives to address cross-cutting issues, Stewart and colleagues (1999) found that most had long histories of concern, ambiguous definitions of the problem, a lack of clarity about goals and uncertainty about cause and effect, and as a result there was a lack of direction to any policies developed. Parsons (1995) argues that much more time needs to be given to clarifying the problem and developing shared definitions and goals than is generally the case. Other studies have suggested that developing a shared broad vision is important in gaining commitment from the wide range of stakeholders necessary to achieve strategic change (Pettigrew et al. 1992). For example, Evans and Killoran (2000) found that having a shared understanding of health inequalities did facilitate change by improving ownership of action. However, in the HAZ experience, political pressures for early wins inhibited the HAZs from taking the time necessary to develop such shared understanding of what they meant by 'health inequalities'.

The HAZs had goals that focused on improving both average health and reducing inequalities in health simultaneously, although with differing relative priority in each HAZ depending on local circumstances. However, a range of commentators have questioned whether it is possible simultaneously to improve average health and to reduce inequalities (Anand 2002; Klein 2003). In fact, it has been suggested that improving average levels of health may actually lead to an increase in health inequalities (Plewis 1998; Macintyre 2001), as discussed below.

Equally problematically, in the HAZs there was a lack of clarity about what goal to aim for when reducing internal inequalities in health. Should the main aim be to raise the floor, that is focus improvements on the most disadvantaged groups, but without necessarily reducing the health divide, or should it explicitly target 'closing the gap', by ensuring that any health improvements were larger or faster among disadvantaged groups than the rest of the population. These different goals in relation to reducing health inequalities within an area require different kinds of intervention strategies. However, until there is more clarity about overall goals, it will be difficult for local partnerships to develop specific strategies.

Nationally, the rhetoric of reducing health inequalities was not matched by the goals and targets that were set, which often focused on averages (Macintyre 2003a), making it difficult to focus on inequalities locally. Even when the national inequalities targets were published (DH 2001b), while these provided significant symbolism of the importance placed on health inequalities, they did not really help to focus local action. For example, stakeholders from North Staffordshire argued that infant mortality was such a rare event locally that it was not easy to use such a target to galvanise local support or to address it. Similar concerns have been expressed in other locations (Benzeval and Meth 2002a; Evans 2003).

Understanding the causes

Since the 1980s understanding of the causes of health inequalities has advanced considerably (Graham 2000a). Nevertheless, further research is required to understand precise cause and effect relationships or the relative importance of different determinants of health across the life course. Moreover, such general knowledge provides information only on plausible rather than efficacious policy options (Macintyre 2003b). The concentration of research on general causes rather than specific interventions means that there is a very limited evidence base about what works to reduce health inequalities (Macintyre 2003b). In so far as such evidence exists, it generally relates to downstream rather than upstream policies (Macintyre 2003a). It was partly in response to this that HAZs were encouraged to innovate with new ways of addressing health inequalities, evaluate their endeavours and disseminate their findings widely.

In the three HAZs, different attempts were made both to draw on the existing evidence base in designing interventions and to evaluate projects to develop evidence about 'what works' further. In addition, efforts were made to synthesise and disseminate the lessons from projects (e.g. Geser 2002; Jacobs et al. 2002) and the broader HAZ experience (e.g. Sheffield First for Health 2002; Vernon et al. 2002). Nevertheless, much more needs to be done in a more systematic and substantive manner to promote further learning about how best to reduce health inequalities locally. For example, there is a need to monitor and evaluate the effect of different social policies on health (Acheson 1998; Exworthy et al. 2003) and to ensure that general intervention studies and routine datasets include sufficient information so that the impact on the distribution of outcomes can be monitored (Macintyre 2003b).

The complex, and sometimes contradictory, nature of the evidence about the causes of health inequalities means that policy makers can often find research to support any approach they want to adopt (Carlisle 2001). Given this, and without a very specific definition of the goal in some HAZs, almost anything could legitimately be defined as a priority. In both East London and North Staffordshire, perhaps for different reasons, there was a sense that the initial HAZ investments, at least, had been a bit of a scatter gun approach. In all three HAZs, concerns were expressed about why particular issues had been supported as part of an inequalities programme. In East London, in particular, given the perception of the universal nature of the problem, everything was considered relevant to health inequalities and hence there had been quite a struggle to agree priorities, and some bitterness among stakeholders that particular issues had or had not been prioritised.

These problems were exacerbated by the initial rounds of HAZ project funding being based on a bidding process so that HAZs had little input into the design of the initiatives. As discussed in Chapter 6, over time HAZs moved to a commissioning process, so that they had more control over the content of the projects to ensure they better met their aims. However, this did not overcome some of the problems associated with the lack of clarity about priorities for tackling health inequalities locally and how these could be met.

Not only was there a lack of clarity about specific interventions to address health inequalities, but also there was often a variety of understandings about the general causes of the problem. In some quarters there was a clear and widespread acceptance of the social model of health, but nowhere was this universal. Nevertheless, the three HAZs did try to address some aspects of the social determinants of health. However, it was difficult to get consideration of health impact on the overcrowded agendas of different LA departments, although each HAZ had some successes in relation to this. For example, in Sheffield, a housing and health initiative had become an integral part of the Housing Department of the City Council and was expanding its role, while in East London a health impact assessment tool had been developed which was in considerable demand from regeneration initiatives.

In addition, there is still some way to go to ensure that there is sufficient understanding that it is the distribution of the determinants of health that needed to be addressed to reduce health inequalities. A number of studies have shown that general efforts to improve services, especially if they rely on individuals accessing them, can actually exacerbate inequalities in health (Petticrew and Macintyre 2001). For example, an income maximisation project, if not targeted carefully, could improve the circumstances of those more affluent rather than those most in need. However, even in regeneration initiatives that do target those most in need, some evidence suggests that the most disadvantaged are often still excluded by the processes that try to target them (Curtis et al. 2002).

Similarly, within the health sector some projects adopted a targeted approach to providing services in relation to need and considered the distributional impact of their activities. However, in other cases, there were services that still very much thought along the lines of 'one size fits all'. There was often considerable political pressure for equal resources per area or per general practitioner (GP) practice rather than in relation to need. The debate about the comparative benefits of universalist versus targeted services is not a new one, and it is an issue that is acknowledged in the 2003 health inequalities strategy (DH 2003c). There was also concern that while the HAZ funded special projects tailored to the particular needs of disadvantaged groups, mainstream services did not see this as a core part of their responsibilities. Yet, often such groups were those most in need, and tailoring services to the needs of particular groups is likely to be a more effective, if perhaps more expensive, way of improving their health, and hence reducing health inequalities (Benzeval and Meth 2002b).

Given this, a key debate in all three HAZs was the extent to which initiatives should be targeted at geographic areas and communities of interest. There was a strong belief among key stakeholders that this ability to invest differentially was crucial in addressing health inequalities, and would not have been possible without the additional ring-fenced resources that the HAZ received.

Health inequalities: a wicked issue in a complex world

The HAZ experience of trying to address health inequalities raised a number of issues in common with the growing literature on addressing complex social problems – so called 'wicked issues' (Clarke and Stewart 1997), which were discussed in Chapter 2. Three sets of issues arising from this literature are important in relation to the HAZs' experience of tackling health inequalities:

- developing local solutions to local problems
- achieving strategic changes in a complex world
- having a dedicated policy space for complex priorities.

Developing local solutions to local problems

The early framework established for HAZs very much emphasized their *raison d'être* as being to develop local strategies to reduce health inequalities in response to local needs (e.g. DH 1997a). Such an approach reflected the growing recognition that addressing complex social problems requires a systems perspective, which in turn needs a new style of governance with much more local autonomy (Clarke and Stewart 1997; Stewart et al. 1999; Chapman 2002). It is argued that central governments need to set clear priorities and boundaries and then allow local agencies to develop their own approaches appropriate to local needs (Chapman 2002). However, in health policy more broadly, while much of the rhetoric emphasizes local flexibility and responsiveness, the NHS has become a much more centrally managed system (Moon and Brown 2000; Chapman 2002). As a result, central–local tensions, endemic in British social policy, have continued as both national and local governments struggle to find new ways of working together (Stewart et al. 1999).

For HAZs there was, initially, the promise of being able to use their resources in innovative ways to respond to local needs, and they were managed against the milestones that they set themselves. There is clear evidence that they set out to try to do this (Judge et al. 1999). However, as time progressed, their performance management regime was made much tighter and refocused on mainstream NHS issues (House of Commons 2002). Not only was the focus of HAZs' performance management changed to reflect central priorities but also the balance of their budgets was altered to contain more earmarked monies, constraining their capacity to respond to local needs. Moreover, even though HAZs initially had considerable flexibility in their own resource use, the agencies that made up their partnerships had to respond to their individual centrally determined priorities, again reducing the actual flexibility of HAZs as part of local systems to address local needs.

The lack of consistency of priorities for different agencies has been highlighted as an inhibiting factor in local efforts to tackle health inequalities in a number of studies (Benzeval and Meth 2002a; Exworthy et al. 2002; Evans 2003). The emphasis on common core targets, including reducing health inequalities, as part of the public service agreements is therefore helpful (DH 2002a). However, given the long-term nature of health inequalities, more needs to be done to embed into mainstream performance assessment systems across different agencies the monitoring of activities to tackle them (Exworthy et al. 2003).

Achieving strategic changes in a complex world

Reducing health inequalities is what Bryson (1988) calls a 'big win' goal, which requires a comprehensive strategy to address it. To achieve this, strategies must be supported by a strong coalition and have a clear vision; the problem must have a clear cause-and-effect relationship, a solution needs to be proposed and resources need to be available to implement it. Without these criteria being fulfilled, a strategy to achieve a 'big win' is likely to fail (Bryson 1988). However, as Clarke and Stewart (1997) argue, 'wicked issues', such as health inequalities, need system-wide action and since it is impossible to predict the consequences of action across complex open systems, it is argued that it is better to try multiple approaches and let the direction emerge over time, learning from 'what works' (Plesk and Greenhalgh 2001; Chapman 2002) – what Bryson (1988) might call a 'small win' approach. To achieve this, organizations need to be capable of adapting through learning (Plesk and Greenhalgh 2001; Chapman 2002). Again, there is evidence that some of this thinking was present in the development and early implementation of HAZs, as described in Chapter 6. For example, there was a strong emphasis on them becoming learning organizations. However, simultaneously they were performance managed very tightly against their early plans, and slippage or deviations were challenged forcefully by the DH and its regional offices. The literature suggests that to achieve 'big wins' in complex systems, having agreed a clear broad vision and systems, the emphasis needs to be on developing a process for improvement and learning (Plesk and Wilson 2001; Chapman 2002). Again, there is evidence that the HAZs did try to do this. For example, North Staffordshire HAZ was concentrating on developing a local toolkit to improve underlying processes for reducing health inequalities, while Sheffield was attempting to ensure that health inequalities and evaluations and learning were much more firmly on local partnership agendas. However, being outside of the mainstream made this difficult for HAZs to achieve. Tackling health inequalities needs to be part of core agendas (DH 2003c) in order for such a systems approach to be more feasible. In addition, there needs to be more of an appreciation of the implications of working in a complex open system for achieving 'big win' goals in 'small win' ways.

Having a dedicated policy space for complex priorities

Stewart and colleagues (1999) note the paradox that while issues often need a specific unit to raise awareness of them, this also marginalises them.

Conversely, drawing them into mainstream agencies can dilute them, reducing their visibility. The policy space that the HAZ initiative created for health inequalities was broadly welcomed locally as it provided an opportunity to focus and think about the problem in ways that would not otherwise have been possible. However, it was also acknowledged that it had proved difficult for HAZs to influence mainstream services in relation to health inequalities. While in part this was because they were seen as 'outside of the system', providing them with very little leverage, it was also a reflection of the more general policy treatment of health inequalities over the same period. As a number of other policy studies of health inequalities have noted, the reality for mainstream agencies was that other 'must dos' had greater priority, thus reducing their capacity to take on board the inequalities agenda (Benzeval and Meth 2002a; Exworthy et al. 2002; Evans 2003).

Within general policy in relation to health inequalities in England it is now clear that this agenda must become part of the mainstream (DH 2003c). However, in doing this it is important that the tension between general objectives and reducing health inequalities is acknowledged and addressed (Exworthy et al. 2003). One more radical counter-argument to this has, however, been put forward by Klein (2003) who suggests that given that social determinants of health are often important social goals in their own right, and that evidence about what to do in relation health inequalities specifically is not clear, there should not be a specific policy in relation to health inequalities. Instead strategies to address other social problems should be pursued and if health inequalities are reduced as a byproduct of these that would be an added bonus. More generally, however, there is significant consensus that addressing health inequalities does require specific action, and hence having this as a policy objective alongside other social goals, is important. At the same time, it is argued that it is important to assess the impact of other social programmes on health inequalities (Acheson 1998; Exworthy et al. 2003), so that learning about how to tackle them can be generated (Macintyre 2003b).

Conclusion

Like many social policy initiatives, HAZs have been neither a total success nor a total failure. The added resources and policy focus on health inequalities enabled local champions associated with HAZ to accelerate some of the necessary processes to build local capacity to address them. In doing so, they also exposed some of the gaps in understanding about how to develop and implement effective local strategies to reduce health inequalities.

The HAZ idea was over-ambitious in its aspiration to reduce health inequalities in a short timescale with limited resources. But it was symbolically important as an early marker of the government's commitment to address health inequalities. HAZs were set up to tackle complex interwoven problems with limited resources, inappropriate timescales and a patchy evidence base about how to do so. They operated in a fast-moving world with a range of different local contexts with differing degrees of local autonomy at different points in time. Nevertheless, they do appear to have given an effective voice to health inequalities locally. Moreover, perhaps what the HAZ experience demonstrates most is that there is no blueprint about how best to address the complex causes of health inequalities at the local level. This does not mean that there should be no further action. Progress can be made in 'small wins' and by learning from different attempts in different contexts. To achieve this, there needs to continue to be a dedicated policy focus on health inequalities at the local level.

Chapter 8

Assessing the impact of Health Action Zones

Linda Bauld, Helen Sullivan, Ken Judge and Jane Mackinnon

One of the slogans adopted by New Labour on the eve of its 1997 election victory was 'What matters is what works' (Davies et al. 2000a). Subsequent government initiatives have either sought to build on existing evidence of effectiveness or have attempted to demonstrate their impact in an effort to contribute to policy learning. Health Action Zones were established with both these objectives in mind. The Department of Health commissioned the national evaluation with a clear expectation that it would collect evidence about the impact of Health Action Zones (DH 1998a).

Several chapters in this volume have already described outcomes from HAZs relating to issues such as partnership working and addressing inequalities. What this chapter does is focus specifically on the issue of measuring impact *based on the views of a range of actors and different types of evidence.* Because of the complexity of HAZs, determining how and where they 'made a difference' is difficult and conclusions drawn from different sources can be conflicting. What this chapter attempts to do, therefore, is to present and discuss potentially competing understandings of impact by drawing on data collected from a range of points of view. The chapter begins with a general discussion regarding the challenge of evaluating impact in relation to complex initiatives. It then summarises findings from three different perspectives:

- an 'external' assessment of overall impact, involving a review of routinely available health data to identify differences between HAZ and non-HAZ areas in relation to key health outcomes
- an 'internal' description of progress and impact from the perspective of project managers in all twenty-six HAZs
- an additional 'internal' view from a wider range of stakeholders in eight HAZs.

Evaluating impact

Gathering evidence about the effectiveness of different treatments and interventions is a routine part of modern science and medicine. But it is only since 2000 that the push to collect such evidence has extended to other policy areas (Davies et al. 2000b; Glendinning et al. 2002). Evidence is now expected to play an important role in influencing decisions about which policies will be developed, and subsequently whether they will be continued or expanded. Various mechanisms have been established to inform evidence-based practice in the United Kingdom including the Cochrane and Campbell Collaborations and the ESRC centres for evidence-based research. In addition specific evaluative tools that aim to improve the identification and assessment of impact have become popular, such as Health and Environmental Impact Assessment instruments. However, it is not always clear what is meant by reference to impact and when evaluators should seek to assess it. Here Chen's (1990) insights are helpful:

> Stakeholders, particularly funding agencies, decision makers, and/or taxpayers, typically want to understand how successful the program is in achieving its purposes and/or through what kinds of causal mechanisms it will operate.
>
> (Chen 1990, p. 143)

In addition, Chen (1990) makes the link between impact and judgements of success about the intervention. This is not necessarily a straightforward relationship but one mediated by the operating context (Pawson and Tilley 1997). For example, in relation to Health Action Zones, the specified purposes of the initiative were ambitious, long term and contingent upon several factors, including the assembly and deployment of appropriate horizontal and vertical collaborative capacity within the zone. Previous chapters have demonstrated the extent of this complexity and the multitude of ways in which different projects, organisations and processes interacted to form the HAZ.

The other element of context that is relevant to any discussion of evaluating the impact of HAZs is the external policy environment. Chapter 4 outlined in some detail how this altered throughout the lifetime of the initiative. The overall aims and programmes of HAZs were forced to shift with a change in ministerial priorities. Budget cuts and, eventually, a truncation of the initiative followed. Evaluator assessments of programme impact in this turbulent context are likely to be modest. As HAZs shifted direction, the evaluation was expected to alter course as well. As we outlined in Chapter 3, the result was that many of the original research questions we devised in 1999 became redundant (or data to attempt to answer them could not be collected) as the initiative developed.

Beyond the specific operating context of any particular initiative, the literature on complex community-based interventions such as HAZs identifies a variety of other factors that can limit the identification and collection of evidence in relation to impact. These include the following:

- *Political factors:* the nature of the political cycle means that governments are frequently unwilling to wait for new policy interventions to 'bed down' before demanding evidence of impact. Similarly as new priorities emerge, initiatives are often required to demonstrate how they will contribute to the delivery of these new priorities often at the expense of their original aims. In the United Kingdom the nature of central–local relations means that the top-down perspective is dominant. This can 'crowd out' the views of other stakeholders whose perspectives on and criteria for positive impact may not be shared with central government (Henry 2002). Proponents of evidence-based practice argue that research and evaluation strategies need to be informed by the perspectives of all key stakeholders (Nutley et al. 2002). However, it is difficult to find examples of such strategies within central government.
- *Technical factors:* the complexity of the relationships associated with meeting cross-cutting goals mean that the causal mechanisms highlighted by Chen (1990) may not easily be established. This is compounded as many of the initiatives are themselves complex, attempting to achieve change in a number of locations from individuals to systems (Connell et al. 1995). Attempts to unravel causal relationships can result in costly evaluation programmes which may not be considered worthwhile investments.
- *Cultural factors:* partly arising from the above, institutions in the United Kingdom are less likely to be persuaded of the value of evaluation (Sanderson 2002). Sanderson (2001) identifies the tendency to 'blame' officials rather than provide the support to address problems as a key cultural factor rendering local government 'antithetical' to a learning culture. This is also evident at central government level, notwithstanding its expressed commitment to evidence based practice. For example, Powell and Exworthy (2001) discuss how central government's design and operation of policy, process and resource streams continues to inhibit rather than facilitates a focus on health inequalities in spite of the availability of evidence about the importance of a 'joined-up' approach.

Consequently local and (to some extent) national bodies are unlikely to put in place planning systems that support the identification of impact in anything other than crude ways.

With these limitations in mind, this chapter attempts to provide some insight into the impact of HAZs from three sources: routine health data, the perspectives of project managers, and the views of a range of HAZ staff and partners in a selection of Health Action Zone areas.

Exploring population level impact

Health Action Zones were expected to make a significant contribution to improving population health and reducing health inequalities in their area. However, relatively little thought was given to how zones or central government would measure whether HAZs had made a difference overall. In contrast to some subsequent policy initiatives, the Department of Health did not require HAZs to collect a common dataset (Bauld et al. 2003). In addition, the national evaluation was not commissioned (or resourced) to use traditional evaluation tools (such as household surveys across HAZs) to measure any changes between baseline and follow-up through time. Efforts were made by the evaluation team in 1999 to work with a range of key allies to identify a common set of core indicators. Several meetings were held with representatives from a range of HAZs but agreement could not be reached. As a result, attempting to measure changes in population health through analysis of common data collected by HAZs is not possible.

Given that there are no HAZ-specific data for measuring the impact of the initiative, it was necessary to identify appropriate routinely collected statistics that could shed some light on changes in population health through time. One of the best sources of this type of data is the *Compendium of Clinical and Health Indicators*, which is commissioned by the Department of Health and produced by the National Centre for Health Outcomes Development (NCHOD). The *Compendium* brings together 150 indicators from several datasets including the Public Health Common Data Set indicators, population health outcome indicators, *Our Healthier Nation* indicators, clinical indicators, cancer survival indicators and others (DH 2003a).

Reviewing the data

We selected a range of indicators from the *Compendium* with the objective of identifying whether there was a demonstrable difference between HAZ and non-HAZ areas in relation to changes in health outcomes through time. At the time of conducting the analysis, the latest available data related to the year 2001/02. We took as the baseline 1997/98 data, the year before the first wave of Health Action Zones was established.

In order to perform the analysis of data in a way that would allow some level of comparison of HAZ and non-HAZ areas the chosen denominator was local authority level data. Local authorities within HAZ areas were compared with those outside HAZ areas with similar levels of disadvantage. Although there are commonly problems with coding and recording systems of health indicators at this level, the fact that the data were drawn from one source meant that they were presented in a consistent way and were therefore comparable through time.

Table 8.1 Average deprivation scores for HAZ and non-HAZ areas

	First wave HAZs (N=32)	Second wave HAZs (N=35)	Deprived non-HAZ LAs (N=67)	Non-deprived LAs (N=220)
Average deprivation score (Indicies of Deprivation 2000)	35.92	33.76	32.83	15.53

Data were analysed for a range of health indicators relevant to HAZ activities. The analysis was conducted in order to obtain the percentage change in each indicator between 1997/98 and the year 2001/02. This was calculated for four groups, local authorities (LAs) in first wave HAZs (N=32) and second wave HAZs (N=35), the most deprived non-HAZ LAs (N=67) and non-deprived non-HAZ LAs (N=220). The percentage change for the whole of England was also calculated for each indicator.

The 67 local authorities associated with HAZs were ranked in the most disadvantaged 134 of the total 354. We compared aggregate indicators for these HAZ LAs with a similar number (67) also in the most disadvantaged group of 134 but not part of HAZs, and with the remaining, more advantaged group of 220 who were also not associated with HAZs.

Table 8.1 highlights the differences in levels of deprivation between the four groups of local authorities. First wave HAZs contained the most deprived LAs followed by second wave HAZs. Deprived non-HAZ areas showed slightly lower levels of deprivation than the HAZ areas. However, the average deprivation score for non-deprived LAs being half that of the other groups clearly demonstrates that these local authority areas were more affluent.

Table 8.2 presents findings relating to mortality from all causes. Data are presented for all age groups and are also split into three age groups to try to gain a clearer picture of any changes that might have taken place.

Table 8.2 illustrates that between 1997 and 2002 the mortality rate for all causes of death decreased in all areas for the population as a whole and for each of the three age groups. The reduction was fairly similar across the four groups of areas, although it was slightly less in the deprived non-HAZ areas. In the under-15 age group, mortality from all causes reduced in each area apart from deprived non-HAZ areas. The largest decrease in child mortality was in non-deprived LAs in non-HAZ areas. All areas showed a decrease in mortality in the 15–64 age group, although deprived non-HAZ areas demonstrated a smaller decrease than HAZ areas and non-deprived local authorities. Mortality amongst older people (65–74) decreased in all areas, with second wave HAZs and non-deprived LAs showing the largest decrease.

Table 8.2 Mortality from all causes in HAZ and non-HAZ areas

Variable	% Change 1997–2001				% Change for England
	First wave HAZs	Second wave HAZs	Deprived non-HAZ LAs	Non-deprived LAs	
All mortality all ages	−8.27	−8.07	−7.72	−8.88	−8.54
All mortality <15	−6.55	−7.09	1.77	−11.63	−7.05
All mortality 15–64	−7.10	−7.12	−4.56	−7.17	−6.71
All mortality 65–74	−13.40	−14.79	−13.46	−15.43	−14.82

Table 8.3 shows that mortality from CHD decreased between 1997 and 2001 in all four groups of areas. The decrease was largest in second wave HAZs for the 15–64 age group. In the 65–74 age group the decrease in non-deprived LAs was greater than that in first and second wave HAZ areas. However, in both age groups the decrease in HAZ areas was greater than that in deprived non-HAZ LAs.

Table 8.3 Changes in health indicators in HAZ and non-HAZ areas

Variable	% Change 1997–2001				% Change for England
	First wave HAZs	Second wave HAZs	Deprived non-HAZ LAs	Non-deprived LAs	
CHD mortality 15–64	−20.38	−22.00	−18.30	−21.49	−20.95
CHD mortality 65–74	−21.87	−20.75	−21.47	−24.84	−23.18
Suicide mortality	−5.50	0.09	5.32	−3.34	−1.09
Mortality from accidental falls	31.34	14.53	17.05	9.06	14.53
Mortality from accidents	0.69	−2.69	−1.38	3.24	0.85

Table 8.3 also shows that the mortality rate from suicide increased in deprived non-HAZ LA areas and in second wave HAZs between 1997 and 2002; with the greatest increase evident in the deprived non-HAZ LA areas. Non-deprived LAs saw a decrease in the mortality rate from suicide between 1997 and 2001 but the greatest decrease was in first wave HAZ areas.

The final two indicators presented in Table 8.3 are measures of mortality from accidents and accidental falls. Mortality from accidental falls increased in all four groups of areas between 1997 and 2002. Mortality rates from accidents also increased in non-deprived LAs and first wave HAZs. The deprived non-HAZ LA group demonstrated a decrease in the mortality rate from accidents, with the greatest decrease evident in second wave HAZs.

Interpreting the differences

A mixed picture emerges from this brief analysis. Between 1997 and 2002, HAZs appear to have outperformed other areas in relation to a number of indicators that are related to their programmes and national policy priorities. First wave HAZs in particular, who had an extra year to make an impact, appear to have seen more positive changes in relation to all cause mortality and CHD mortality than other areas. Findings are however not consistent between indicators. Mortality from suicide increased in all areas, with the largest increase in first wave HAZs. This is despite the existence of some HAZ programmes focussing on addressing the causes of suicide, particularly amongst young men. In addition, second wave HAZs and deprived non-HAZ local authorities saw a decrease in mortality and accidents from falls, while all other areas increased. This is despite the fact that several first wave HAZs had projects with an accident prevention focus.

Given this mixed picture, it is worth considering the role of routinely available statistics of this kind in drawing any conclusions about the impact of a complex initiative such as HAZs. Caution in interpreting findings must be exercised, for at least three reasons. The first of these relates to the long-term nature of population health change. The second concerns problems with grouping areas and drawing conclusions about differences between them. Finally, any review of routine data of this kind must acknowledge the difficulties associated with attributing change to a particular intervention.

Population health change is a long-term endeavour, and changes such as reductions in CHD mortality are achieved only through concerted efforts over a number of years. The research team could access only data that related to the relatively short period 1997–2002. It may be that any contribution made by HAZs to some of the indicators selected will be realised only over the longer term. This is particularly the case when, as with many HAZs, projects were specifically aimed at children and families. A recent review of the evidence base for community health initiatives revealed uncertainty about the efficacy of many interventions, and limited knowledge about the longer term impact of such interventions (Bauld et al. 2001b). Often this is because of the same types of issues that affected the HAZ evaluation and HAZs themselves – lack of satisfactory baseline data and a short lifespan. In many cases an initiative has ended and the political cycle has moved on just when data to evaluate its impact becomes available.

A second reason for caution in interpreting Tables 8.2 and 8.3 relates to the way that the data are presented. In order to compare differences between HAZs and other parts of England we grouped first and second wave HAZs and other local authority areas, differentiating between those that were more or less deprived. While this does highlight contrasts, it masks the huge range of variation between areas. There is little doubt that in relation to accident prevention, for instance, some HAZs invested more in addressing this issue. Likewise areas outside of HAZs may have had particular interventions aimed at reducing accidents. Our work and that of others has shown how widely local contextual factors can vary and how difficult it often is to directly compare different areas (Mackenzie et al. 2001b).

Finally, in describing changes in population health between areas it is important to consider the issue of attribution. By merely collecting and reviewing routinely available statistics we have no way of determining whether the changes observed are due to HAZ activities or have been caused by other factors. Other studies have demonstrated how efforts to address particular health problems in one area can often be mirrored in neighbouring areas as policies develop (Nutbeam et al. 1993; Platt et al. 2003). In addition, initiatives with similar aims can often be implemented in the same areas, confounding an effect from a single intervention. As HAZs are amongst the most deprived areas in England, this has made them the focus of a wide range of initiatives such as the New Deal for Communities and Sure Start. These often share a number of cross-cutting themes and are aimed at tackling the broad agenda of inequalities. It would therefore be very difficult, if not impossible, to differentiate at a population level between the success attributable to HAZ or another initiative.

Earlier, Chen's (1990) description of what is meant by reference to impact highlighted the importance of establishing causal links to assess the success of an intervention. The exploration of population health data will not help to unravel complex causal relationships, either within a single initiative such as HAZ, or when trying to disentangle a number of initiatives and attribute success to one alone. A theory-based approach to evaluation, described in previous chapters, attempts to identify these links in order to improve efforts to attribute particular outcomes to specific interventions. But this process has its own limitations, and there is therefore still a place for reviewing routinely available data at the national level. An analysis of such data can be used to give a broad view of the health of the population, if only to demonstrate that changes have taken place and to provide some context for more in-depth local analysis of what HAZs have achieved. We now turn to local evidence of impact, from the perspective of those working in Health Action Zones.

Project managers' perceptions

In addition to 'objective' measures of impact such as measuring changes in routine data, more subjective accounts of HAZ achievements provide another means of assessing outcomes. As Chapter 4 outlined, key informants throughout the evaluation were local leaders of the initiative – project managers – in each of the twenty-six HAZs. Their views regarding the achievements of their HAZ were routinely sought. Perceptions of general progress in the six months preceding each interview were explored, as well as views regarding progress in relation to specific issues, such as achieving HAZ principles.

Overall progress

Initial interviews with project managers in 1999 revealed a great deal of enthusiasm for the HAZ initiative. Interviewees were almost universally optimistic about the early steps that had been taken to implement projects and work towards achieving longer term objectives (Judge et al. 1999). The challenge, as one respondent described it, was to sustain this optimism:

> I think it's going to be maintaining the enthusiasm ... that's got to be sustained because we're talking here about seven to ten years ... and that enthusiasm and drive has got to continue and it's got to come from something which is a project into the mainstream.

Figure 8.1 shows project managers' responses on a five-point scale when asked to rate the progress of their HAZ in the six months leading up to each interview. As the figure illustrates, project managers' views regarding overall progress changed as the initiative developed.

When project managers were asked to rate the overall progress in their HAZ in 2000, responses given by project managers were quite positive. The majority said that 'a great deal of' or 'good' progress had been made. Perceptions of progress were also fairly positive in 2001. However, it is clear from Figure 8.1 that project managers in spring 2002 were less confident about the amount of progress their HAZ had been able to make in the previous six months.

When questioned further about their views regarding progress, managers highlighted a number of issues. On the positive side, they appeared confident that the 'HAZ way of working' was being adopted by a range of local agencies. This was described as the 'added value' of the HAZ, manifested

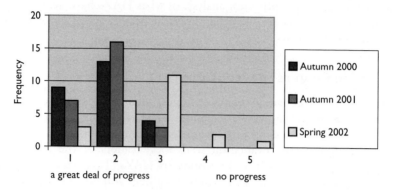

Figure 8.1 Project manager's perceptions of the progress of their HAZ

as giving organisations and individuals the opportunity to do things differently.

The majority of project managers reported that considerable progress had been made in building partnerships within their HAZ. In some areas, partnership working between statutory agencies was described as traditionally weak, and so a considerable amount of effort had been invested locally to improve it. Some also reported that initial enthusiasm for partnerships had been maintained:

> I also measure my success by the level of enthusiasm for the HAZ, I saw that level of enthusiasm when I came here and I think whilst it ebbs and flows at times, it's still there ... that's my intangible measure of how much we've actually achieved.

As Chapter 4 outlined, there were a number of changes in 2001 and 2002 that impacted on the development of the HAZ initiative. One of the most significant was organisational change within the NHS and its partner organisations (DETR 2001; DH 2001d). Some project managers highlighted that a great deal of progress had been made in linking with the newly emerging organisations. They described an increased understanding of the HAZ agenda and how it could contribute to new developments. There was also a higher degree of local ownership of this agenda in some areas, which was seen as a beneficial shift. Although the organisational changes had caused some disruption, many project managers in 2002 saw them as a positive step, as one explained:

> It's also an opportunity to make sure that the HAZ agenda is firmly embedded in the new systems and processes.

Some potential barriers to progress were experienced by HAZs during 2001 and 2002. From the perspective of project managers, the main one was the uncertain climate in which HAZs were operating in relation to continued funding of the initiative. For many HAZs this uncertainty has made planning very difficult. Some project managers said that it had affected their capacity to be 'innovative' and to try new approaches.

In other HAZs, in contrast, project managers reported that they had tried to channel the uncertainty regarding future funding in a positive direction by focussing on convincing partner organisations that they should fund HAZ projects or programmes in the longer term:

> The uncertainty about the future hangs over us all the time. So we can't plan on a longer term basis ... that's been good in some ways because it's made us much more focussed on mainstreaming as an approach to change.

Progress towards HAZ principles

When the creation of HAZs was first announced, ministers set out seven underlying principles for the initiative (DH 1997b). These were described in Chapter 1. Each HAZ was asked to reflect these values in their plans and activities. They were:

- achieving equity
- engaging communities
- working in partnership
- engaging front-line staff
- taking an evidence-based approach
- developing a person-centred approach to service delivery
- taking a whole systems approach.

In the autumn of 2001 project managers were asked to give their personal assessment of the progress made to date in relation to each of the principles listed above. Responses were given on a five-point scale. The average score for responses relating to all seven principles was calculated. Results are shown in Figure 8.2.

Figure 8.2 suggests that, on the whole, project managers felt that good progress had been made towards promoting the seven underpinning principles of HAZs. Most responses – seventeen out of twenty-six – were in the middle of the scale. However, when responses regarding progress towards individual principles were examined in more detail, it was apparent that managers were more positive about some than others. The principles that received the most positive response overall were *working in partnership* and *taking a whole systems approach*.

When asked to explain why they had rated progress towards these principles particularly highly, project managers pointed to the fact that a

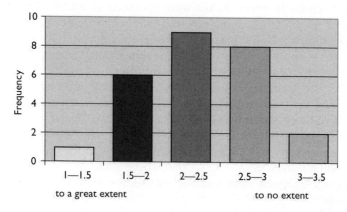

Figure 8.2 Average scores for the seven underpinning HAZ principles across all twenty-six HAZs

considerable amount of time and effort had been put into the development of existing and new partnership arrangements. As previous chapters have outlined, partnerships were operating successfully and were described as the foundation for HAZ work. This positive view of partnership was identified during each round of interviews with project managers, from 1999 to 2002. For instance in 1999, first wave managers pointed out that in addition to partnership working being a long-term goal in its own right, it was also an important means to achieving the goals of the HAZ (Judge et al. 1999). Some interviewees emphasised the importance of building on existing relationships between agencies that were already strong but would benefit from further development. For instance in Sandwell the HAZ programme evolved, at least in part, from the work of Healthy Sandwell 2000, a partnership between local agencies that had been in existence for more than a decade. New partnerships would also help HAZs achieve their long-term strategic goals by building relationships between agencies and forming new networks. Some first wave interviewees highlighted HAZ status as a stimulus for addressing poor relationships between key players. Interviewees also reported that efforts and investments had been made to develop the infrastructure for partnership working.

Likewise in the interviews of autumn 2000, all project managers identified partnership within the HAZ as a 'positive driver for change'. Those interviewed in spring 2002 gave similar views. By 2002, project managers were highlighting partnerships as a key mechanism for mainstreaming HAZ ways of working, and felt that the HAZ had been a useful tool in generating joint working between statutory agencies. As one stated:

> The fact the director of public health post is a joint appointment between PCT and local authority is an example. Public health is now being seen as a shared agenda ... and [this] has been greatly helped by the HAZ.

Thus, at the descriptive level, successive rounds of interviews across all twenty-six HAZs identified partnership working as one of the successes of the initiative. The picture is of course more complex than that, and difficulties were encountered in many areas. This issue is addressed in more detail in Chapter 5.

Project managers identified several of the other underpinning principles of HAZ as more problematic. Fewer positive responses were obtained when they were asked about progress relating to *engaging frontline staff*. Project managers felt that staff in key organisations within the NHS and local government were still not aware of, or involved in, HAZ work. This echoes findings from a report produced by the London HAZs (Vernon et al. 2002). This report highlighted, among other issues, the importance of engaging frontline staff through personal development and providing them with the skills to act as 'agents of change'.

Finally, project managers reported that the issue of progress towards *achieving equity* was difficult to assess. When we discussed the issue with managers in the autumn of 2001, all agreed that it was too early to speculate to what extent HAZs had made any real contribution to saving lives or really addressing inequalities. In terms of *taking an evidence-based approach*, responses were also mixed, but project managers did point out that systems had been put in place to develop the existing (often limited) evidence-base. Some felt that these had been absent earlier in the life of the HAZ initiative.

A fair opportunity?

Project managers views of progress in relation to key elements of the HAZ initiative were relatively positive from 1999 to 2002. However, given the changing policy context we asked managers in the spring of 2001 and 2002: '*Do you think your HAZ has been given a fair opportunity to realise its potential?*' Results are shown in Figure 8.3.

As Figure 8.3 shows, opinions amongst project managers were mixed regarding whether HAZs had been given a fair opportunity to realise their potential. Overall, project managers were more optimistic in 2001 than 2002. When asked to explain their responses in the spring of 2002, a dominant theme was that mixed messages from the centre around long-term aims of the HAZ and the consequent pressure for quick wins had been a source of ongoing frustration. Other key themes touched on similar issues identified by the case study components of the evaluation (described in Chapters 5–7). These themes included:

- scale and nature of the problems HAZs were to tackle
- HAZs realised potential, but within the constraints of a short-term initiative

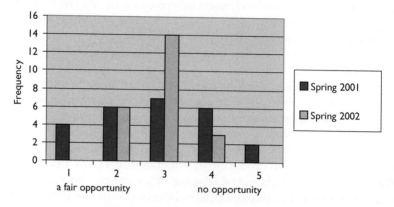

Figure 8.3 Project managers' perceptions of whether HAZs were given a fair opportunity to realise their potential

- impact of changing national policy
- local versus national priorities
- uncertainty of funding.

Some project managers felt that HAZs had not been able to realise their potential due to the nature of the problems that need to be tackled:

> Health and inequalities are about what people eat and whether or not they have got a job and what their educational attainment is and the kinds of houses they live in ... we are talking about the root causes of health, not about giving existing services some additional capacity. So from that point of view, we haven't been given a fair opportunity.

Others were more realistic about the original aims of HAZs and in that context felt that the initiative had contributed to positive change:

> It [the HAZ initiative] has contributed to a whole range of interventions to tackle inequality in its broader sense and from that point of view I think it is very much to be applauded. However, I think if you really want to have a vehicle for tackling health inequalities then HAZs would have to be around for another 25 years at least.

Some felt HAZ should have been allowed to stick to their original plans rather than adhere to new ministerial priorities, as this caused some disruption to progress:

> I think if we had been allowed to do what we set out to do and to stick broadly to the programme we set out to deliver ... the collective HAZs could have achieved a great deal more than we have done.

Some project managers highlighted differences between national and local level in relation to the opportunities available. They argued that organisations at the local level had been more sympathetic:

> Locally I would say yes, there have been very few barriers to doing what we needed to do. Instead [we've received] a lot of support and it came at the right time. Nationally I would have to say there have been problems in allowing us to reach our potential.

Finally, in 2002, project managers commented on how HAZs had been 'overtaken' by more recent developments and initiatives, such as Neighbourhood Renewal and NHS reconfiguration, and consequently had not been able to maintain their status or realise their full potential:

> I think if we were given another three and a half years with some organisational stability and a stable set of partners we might have a better chance of demonstrating success and impact.

Learning from HAZs

Chapter 4 summarised the policy developments leading to the development of Local Strategic Partnerships and Primary Care Trusts. By 2002 these new partnerships were in place in most parts of England and HAZ project managers were actively working to influence their development. A series of policy documents, beginning with the *NHS Plan* in 2000, had made it clear that HAZ 'learning' was to be transferred to PCTs and LSPs and that the new organisations were to assume responsibility for key elements of the HAZ programme (DH 2000c, 2001d). As we outlined in Chapter 4, project managers suggested that, by 2002, HAZs were already working with PCTs and LSPs in a number of ways.

In order to determine whether project managers felt that they were being successful in their attempts to pass on lessons from HAZs, we asked them to what extent they felt that learning was being transferred to the LSP? They were asked an identical question relating to PCTs. Results from both questions are presented in Figure 8.4.

As Figure 8.4 outlines, most project managers were optimistic that lessons from HAZ were being transferred, particularly to LSPs. When asked to explain their responses, a variety of reasons were given.

First, project managers were realistic about the future of their HAZ, recognising that policy and organisational changes had occurred that meant the initiative's role had evolved through time. They had come to see LSPs and PCTs as a vehicle for continuing some of the work HAZs had initiated. As one interviewee stated: 'We see the HAZ role very much as supporting other partnerships to be sustainable.'

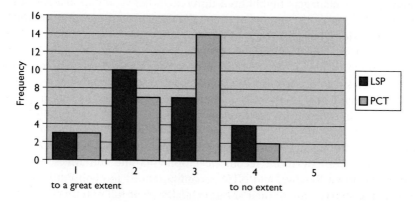

Figure 8.4 Extent to which project managers felt that learning from HAZs was being transferred to LSPs and PCTs

Secondly, there was a belief that the HAZ experience of partnership working at the local level was influencing the structure and processes of LSPs. Similarly, mechanisms to engage community groups or specific community involvement training materials or frameworks were being adopted by both LSPs and PCTs. Other areas in which project managers felt that HAZs could contribute to these new organisations included transferring learning about project monitoring and performance management.

Project managers described their efforts to disseminate lessons learned and provide examples of good practice. Specific efforts to transfer learning included:

- HAZ conferences or learning events targeted at PCTs or LSPs
- publication or circulation of findings from local evaluation
- nominating or supporting key individuals who had worked with the HAZ into positions of leadership within new local partnerships
- commissioning or compiling specific pieces of work – such as population needs assessments – that would feed into the work of new partnerships, particularly PCTs
- working with key HAZ partners, particularly community groups, to assist them in engaging with changing structures.

Thus from the perspective of project managers, there was considerable optimism in 2001 and 2002 regarding HAZ efforts to transfer learning to PCTs and LSPs. It remains to be seen to what extent these new organisations will be influenced in the longer term by the legacy of Health Action Zones.

Local evidence of impact

While project managers' views provide valuable insights into the progress made by HAZs, a wider range of opinions is required to obtain a fuller picture of the impact of the initiative at the local level. The evaluation team worked fairly intensively with a range of case study HAZs, as previous chapters have shown. There were, however, ten zones that did not serve as case studies. Conscious that part of the evaluation was intended to look across all HAZs, project managers were approached in these ten areas in 2002 to ask whether they would participate in work examining impact at the local level (Sullivan et al. 2004). Eight of these HAZs were able to participate. To begin the work, project managers were asked to consult with their colleagues and identify three examples of local 'successes' realised by the HAZ. Each area was then visited to learn more about these examples. Limiting the examples to three proved difficult for some HAZs, but we sought to include all the examples cited. In each HAZ the project manager and those responsible for the 'successful' initiatives were interviewed. Where possible we also interviewed key partners and local evaluators and examined local evaluation material.

The analysis of findings drew upon the theories of change framework described in detail in Chapter 3. We tried to identify the links between the interventions identified as successes, the rationale for these interventions and the observed outcomes. This approach included four steps:

1   Identifying a number of interventions/activities/processes that were described as 'successful' in each HAZ.
2   Examining these to establish what rationales were given for them and how far they were justified as part of a wider HAZ strategy.
3   Exploring why each intervention was described as successful, including the kind of evidence that was given to justify this success.
4   Considering how far these interventions were viewed as successful locally by reference to the evidence presented of success and its limits.

Identifying local success

In total thirty-four interventions were highlighted as examples of 'success' by the eight case study HAZs (Sullivan et al. 2004). These are categorised in Box 8.1 in terms of: the prime focus of the intervention (such as service development); the targeting of a particular population or group; interventions in relation to a specific disease; or to promote local learning.

As Box 8.1 shows, most of the locally identified successes (sixteen) were service related and focused on children and families or employment. Ten focussed on a particular population group such as older people. Only two were disease focused and both of these reflected national priorities. The six learning interventions were very varied, including the development of new techniques such as Health Impact Assessment and the application of new ways of working such as whole systems events and stakeholder evaluation. One of the interesting characteristics of the examples of success provided is that they cover such a wide range of different types of activity. They cut across many of the main programme areas identified by HAZs in their

Box 8.1 Successful HAZ initiatives

Service (16)	**Population/group** (10)
Employment (3)	Young people
Children and family support (4)	Community participation (3)
Healthy schools	Smoking cessation
Welfare advice (2)	Ethnic minorities (2)
Voluntary sector development (2)	Older people (2)
Outreach services – mental health	Sexual and reproductive
Healthy Living Centres	health
Minor ailments – pharmacy scheme	
Intermediate care	**Learning** (6)
Disease (2)	Health Impact Assessment (2)
Pulmonary rehabilitation	Stakeholder evaluation
Cancer	Geographic Information
	Systems (GIS)
	Education and training
	Whole Systems Events

implementation plans and described in Chapter 4. This suggests that HAZs were not generally more or less successful at doing particular things, but that local circumstances and priorities probably combined with national factors to influence which particular strands of work were best developed in particular HAZs.

Rationale for action

Establishing the rationale for specific interventions requires those involved to articulate why and how the proposed activity will lead to predetermined outcomes. Rationales for local successes in the eight HAZs ranged from those that were both instinctive and intuitive to those that were supported by material evidence. For instance, in Bury and Rochdale a project to promote change in health services for Black and minority ethnic communities was described as a natural area for HAZ investment because, as one interviewee said, 'everyone knows that service take-up among Black and minority ethnic groups is poor'.

Alternatively, specific evidence was cited by interviewees to explain HAZ activities. In Cornwall and the Isles of Scilly a pulmonary rehabilitation programme was based on project workers' access to evidence about the impact of such programmes in the United States. Elsewhere project rationale was derived from a close examination of the local context. In Wolverhampton, for instance, an employment scheme was based upon a long-term assessment of recruitment and retention problems in the NHS combined with an appreciation of the nature of long-term unemployment in the area.

While those working within the HAZ found it fairly easy to provide a rationale for individual interventions, they found it more difficult to establish links between them and wider HAZ strategy. In some cases this may have been because the links between initiative success and improved health or reduced health inequalities were perceived as self-evident. In other cases it may have been because individuals involved in specific activities were not aware of overall HAZ strategy and saw it as someone else's job to make the links between their specific contribution and wider goals.

Another important factor explaining this difficulty in linking rationales for individual interventions with overall HAZ goals was the relative instability of many HAZ strategies over time. In a minority of cases this was due to local factors, such as problems with partnership working between agencies or lack of local capacity. However, the most pronounced instability was prompted by national changes. These included the development of National Service Frameworks (NSFs) that acted to interrupt the implementation of some agreed strategies as one interviewee explained:

> I know that some aspects of the implementation plan have probably changed dramatically, if I think about the primary care and community services programme … it pretty quickly moved into the big focus on elder care and intermediate care. I think it did that because they had good contacts and effectively guessed the NSF pretty well and those programme activities fitted … the NSF just absolutely brilliantly.

As previous chapters have argued, the biggest interruption to HAZ strategy implementation came with national policy changes and persistent uncertainty about the role and priority of HAZ within the Department of Health from 2000 (Bauld et al. 2001a). This uncertainty affected the life of projects and in some cases resulted in their wholesale removal from the programme. In some places the uncertainty meant that staff left and it was difficult to recruit new people for short-term contracts. Interviewees reported that the perceived lack of national political commitment to HAZ meant that senior figures in localities also became less oriented towards HAZ and gravitated instead to initiatives where the opportunities to make an impact were greater.

Evidence of success

For individual HAZs definitions of success were complex comprising a number of elements, some of which reflected national emphases and others which were derived from local experience and/or individual perspectives. We explored the types of evidence or criteria that local actors used to determine why particular interventions were seen as successful. A range of evidence was used, from more traditional proof of outcomes to qualitative or anecdotal information.

In most of the eight areas, *measurable indicators of success* were cited as being important in defining 'successful' HAZ projects. For example in the Tyne and Wear HAZ minor ailments pharmacy scheme, it was possible for the project to measure the take-up of the scheme by monitoring the number of members of the public who having received a leaflet about the scheme presented that leaflet at their pharmacy. It was also possible to work out how much individual users had saved by accessing the scheme rather than going through their GPs. However, there was widespread recognition that very often the kinds of things that were easily measurable were not particularly good indicators of success in terms of public health. So in one HAZ a community food initiative was measured in relation to how many food co-operatives were established and how many people benefited from one or other of the project elements, rather than in relation to whether the quality of nutrition had improved. Similarly a project that sought to keep older people warm in winter through the use of grants for insulation and home improvements was assessed in terms of how many people had used the scheme rather than any subsequent assessment of changes to their quality of life. This focus on outputs rather than outcomes was reflective of the level of resources generally made available to undertake impact assessment.

There was also concern that definitions of local success should *include process issues* rather than solely focus on the achievement of key health outcomes. One example comes from Wakefield HAZ. Here the development of a cross-sector strategic partnership was considered vitally important in supporting the emergence of a strategic capacity for health in the area that could be sustained through the emergent Local Strategic Partnership. In Brent the use of HAZ resources to support the development of a local voluntary sector umbrella organisation was described as key to providing a means of sustaining a voice for voluntary and community organisations once the HAZ programme had ended.

Linked to this was the identification of success through the adoption of *new ways of thinking and working*. HAZs invested in specific interventions to bring this about such as Tyne and Wear's use of 'whole systems' events to redesign services, including those for 'children with complex needs'. Here the use of a deliberate strategy to change ways of working was described as beneficial by one local worker:

> for children aged 0–5, you have got about 20 key workers, link workers. Immediately a child is diagnosed with complex needs they are part of that joint agency assessment and care planning process rather

than gradually being picked up by this part of the system or that part of the system.

Elsewhere new ways of working emerged in rather less formal ways. For example in Wolverhampton the young people's workstream was able to work with the local housing department to develop a new approach to 'failed tenancies' by young people. This involved the housing department working with other organisations at 'Base 25' a one-stop shop for young people, in order to support young people in their accommodation, rather than responding once the tenancy had failed.

Very often *qualitative material* was considered to be more interesting and telling about the impact of an intervention than hard facts and figures. One example was the pulmonary rehabilitation project in the Cornwall and the Isles of Scilly. Here anecdotal information suggested that clients were using less medication and seeing their GP less because they were able to understand and manage their condition better. In addition, stories told by recipients of the 'community grants' scheme in Wolverhampton of how the funding had provided them with new opportunities were presented as important indicators of how low cost interventions could make an impact.

For local HAZ staff and workers in partner organisations, an important element of HAZ success was its potential *contribution over the long term.* They argued that to affect the kinds of change HAZ was designed for required long-term commitment from a range of local agencies. In several HAZs, examples of success included how individual interventions were expanded and adopted by partner organisations. In one HAZ the success of a benefits take-up project resulted in longer term funding being secured through Neighbourhood Renewal Funding. Elsewhere the success of the pulmonary rehabilitation project was augmented by the establishment of a free-standing, community-organised patients' group which met monthly and was affiliated to the British Lung Foundation.

Assessing success in HAZs

In addition to outlining the type of evidence they had used to define successful interventions, HAZ staff and other local professionals also described what individual projects and processes had achieved. These achievements were closely related to the overall principles or objectives of Health Action Zones that we discussed earlier with reference to project manager's views. The list of achievements included:

- introducing a non-medical perspective to health
- getting important health-related issues onto local agendas
- encouraging closer working relationships between health and social services

- creating infrastructure for sustainable partnership working
- precipitating a culture/attitude shift via the 'HAZ way of working'
- facilitating change to/introduction of mainstream services
- stimulating the involvement of 'the public' as citizens and users
- facilitating shared learning
- enabling experimentation.

First, as we outlined in Chapter 7, some successful HAZ activities were cred-ited with introducing a non-medical perspective to health. HAZ stimulated debate amongst all stakeholders about 'what it means to be healthy' and was described as challenging the dominant 'medical model' of health through the introduction of 'social perspectives'. As one professional described:

> It has enabled a wide diversity of stakeholders, from Jo Public to the voluntary and community sector to mental health services through to children's services to PCT to be involved in this debate about public health and health promotion from a non-medicalised perspective.

Likewise HAZ activities were described as contributing to raising the profile of important health-related issues and getting them onto the agenda of a range of local agencies. Here HAZ was often cited as playing the role of 'champion', profiling issues or the needs of groups that in other circum-stances may have been marginalised. Examples included homeless young people, domestic violence and travellers. In addition to projects enabling vulnerable groups to receive improved support, HAZ also facilitated links with partners outside health and in some cases helped to secure the profile of these issues/groups in developing community strategies.

HAZ activities were also credited with achieving a range of local changes that related to improved relationships between agencies and improved ways of working. This included encouraging closer working relationships between health and social services. This was particularly significant when it involved aspects of both services that had traditionally not worked together. For example, in Hull and East Riding HAZ an intermediate care pro-gramme for elderly people was described as resulting in the improvement of both services and relationships between health and social care. According to one worker the existence of HAZ and the money it brought enabled profes-sionals to imagine alternatives to conventional services and to see how they could benefit at the same time:

> The approach to intermediate care for elderly people was originally not seen as relevant to the acute trust, it was seen as social services type of service. Their consultants just wanted more money spent on hospital beds, but when they saw it began to work, it did have an influence. The acute trust completely revolutionised their whole approach to

access, rapid assessment, they redesigned in building terms the ground floor and ... they saw that success ... was achieved by working across sectors in genuine joint ways.

In addition, as findings in Chapter 5 highlighted, HAZ was credited with preparing the ground for lasting partnership working in each area. Professionals argued that HAZ provided the necessary infrastructure/framework for co-ordinating the activities of a range of organisations. HAZ impact here was important both in terms of creating effective mechanisms for delivering changes in relation to health and in some cases in providing a template for the development of Local Strategic Partnerships. It did this by providing the practical means of partnership engagement:

> Everybody needs to know who their partner is. You need a forum within which to deal. HAZ has simply provided that forum in the absence of anything else.

HAZ activities were also described as helping to create an awareness of the factors that helped to make partnerships work and those which were destructive. For example in one of the eight HAZs there was a need to address specific conflicts before partnership working could become meaningful:

> We have had one or two rough patches ... notably the continuing care criteria where for one reason or another we believed that what the health authority was proposing wasn't deliverable and said we wouldn't sign up under any circumstances. We had to bring in some outside help to get that one sorted out. At the end of the day we actually got an agreement that everybody could sign up to and it has actually worked ... Funnily enough, there was a huge row but it started better working. And in a sense HAZ gave us the elbow room to begin to trust one another and develop again.

HAZ was cited as instrumental in changing the way in which key players related to each other. This was described as leading to a culture or attitude shift. Several professionals referred to long-standing tensions between health authorities and local authorities and the contribution made by HAZ to overcoming these. In one area, for instance, there was:

> a tendency, an awful corrosiveness to speak disparagingly of parties not present and I think that this was not just in the health service here but was a wider feature [through HAZ] I think we were able to see a more grown-up way of working and nowadays those comments are rarely uttered and when they are whoever utters them is made to feel uncomfortable for having done so.

These changed relationships in turn were described as contributing to the emergence of a 'HAZ way of working', an acknowledgement that changing health outcomes was a collective endeavour and that innovation could emerge from cross-sectoral interaction rather than officials 'thinking in their narrow professional boxes'. Testament to the culture change wrought by HAZ was the fact that a wide range of partners continued to attend HAZ co-ordinating meetings even though there might not be any immediate benefit for them:

> So you get 25, 30 people there quite regularly and they are not all Social Services and PCTs and partnership trusts ... there is a whole broad range ... this the value that HAZ has had for us, it has brought people together, it has got people thinking in new ways, doing things in new ways.

Another achievement that was described was a change to mainstream services in several of the eight HAZs. Professionals argued that service delivery had been influenced by HAZ projects or processes. Examples included: the development of a multi-agency strategy for the education and training of health professionals in Leicester HAZ; the use of HAZ funds to support developments in services for older people in Bury and Rochdale HAZ that were subsequently embraced within the National Service Framework; and the stimulation of a locality-wide tobacco strategy in Hull and East Riding arising from a successful local smoking cessation scheme. In some cases these changes were described as a HAZ contribution to the modernisation of mainstream services – this was particularly relevant as modernisation was intended to be one of the underpinning principles of the initiative as a whole.

Successful HAZ projects and activities also stimulated the involvement of 'the public' as citizens and service users. HAZ gave key service providers the means to test out how to involve service users and local communities. In some cases this meant targeting a very specific group, such as Leicester HAZ's involvement of school children in the development of a peer education project for health and Wakefield HAZ's contribution to an estate-based local community and learning centre. In other cases it could mean trying to develop a locality-wide infrastructure such as Brent HAZ's community and voluntary sector development work which supported the development of a system of community representation on the emerging Local Strategic Partnership.

Successful HAZ activities were also credited with facilitating shared learning locally. Learning was highlighted in relation to two themes in particular: learning about the difficulties associated with working in partnership and identifying ways to overcome these, and learning about 'what works' in terms of service change and innovation. For one worker, effective learning required co-operation from all levels of HAZ, not just those involved in projects:

> I think what we have developed is a much more open learning culture, where people don't feel afraid to stand up and say 'well this didn't work but this is why and I'm telling you so you don't go through the same process' ... I think you need to demonstrate that from the top ... so I think we've had to stand up and say 'this hasn't worked and this is why but we're embracing the learning from it' and that enables others to do the same.

Finally, HAZ enabled experimentation. The development of particular projects and activities was considered to have granted local partners the 'freedom to act'. HAZ funding provided an opportunity to try new things without having to demonstrate how they contributed to overall organisational objectives or national targets. This was particularly the case in the first few years of HAZ funding. The resources provided were described as a safety net, meaning that local actors believed that existing services and practices would not necessarily be jeopardised if the HAZ experiment failed.

Limits to success

Notwithstanding these assessments of success, the HAZ staff and others in the eight areas were quick to point out that the potential impact of HAZ had been limited in numerous and often significant ways. Many of the problems they described were similar to those outlined by project managers in all twenty-six zones and highlighted in previous chapters.

Perhaps the most commonly cited constraint was *uncertainty about funding and the future*. This was a common complaint. The perceived failure of the Department of Health to maintain its commitment to significant long-term funding for HAZ combined with the annual uncertainty about how much HAZ money would be made available meant that individual HAZs were limited in their ambitions, not least because they were unable to make or sustain significant investments over time. In the words of one professional, 'one of the problems is that you can't put things in place until you know you've got the funding and then half the year is gone'.

This financial uncertainty was combined with perceived *pressure to meet targets*. The early demands for evidence of 'quick wins' from the centre coupled with the specification of key targets for CHD, mental health and cancer were cited by some as reducing the room for manoeuvre in delivering locally appropriate HAZ interventions.

From 2001 onwards, HAZs like all parts of the health service faced considerable *organisational turbulence*. The 'modernisation' programmes of both the NHS and local government that followed the introduction of HAZ resulted in considerable restructuring of local organisations and the introduction of new posts and people. For some HAZs this was considered critically destabilising. As one manager explained:

> There are three health authorities and eleven primary care groups and even the NHS trusts, every one of these organisations within the past six months would have gone through some sort of organisational tur- bulence. That means a focus on their internal organisations, on people looking at what their own jobs are going to be. I think that every one of our local authorities will now have had a change of chief executive or the impact of cabinet structure of even an elected Mayor. All of these things can have quite a dramatic impact on the people who are our main partners and therefore their ability to focus on partnership working.

Often as a result of this external process of change, HAZs experienced a *loss of interest of key people*. The declining profile of HAZ and the reduced funding it attracted meant that 'people voted with their feet' and sought other more profitable avenues to pursue their objectives. The costs associ- ated with partnership working (even where it was successful) meant that partners assessed their involvement carefully and where perceived benefits were perceived to be low or better elsewhere HAZ was marginalised.

Amongst a minority of professionals in the eight areas we visited, *feelings of isolation* were also reported. In some HAZs participants felt that they had little knowledge of what was going on in the HAZ outside of their own project. Consequently they did not feel linked to a 'bigger picture' and so felt less able to capitalise on the opportunities presented by HAZ such as broadening their networks. In such cases HAZ could become just about money:

> I knew what it [HAZ] was and what it meant to do but I didn't know of any specific projects other than me. I have very little contact. I had no communication. I was just grateful for the funding.

An additional constraint was described as *the role of the centre*. While some HAZ staff felt that the central team within the Department of Health tasked with supporting the initiative had been helpful and constructive, many argued that policy staff had not done enough to try and provide a stable framework within which HAZs could operate. The centre was criticised for requiring HAZs to commit to targets too early so reducing their local flexi- bility and then moving the goal posts altogether when central priorities changed. In addition to limiting the impact of HAZ locally, the centre was also criticised by some for not distilling the key messages from all twenty-six

HAZs on a regular basis and communicating these to other relevant departments. For one manager this situation was more lamentable given the
amount of monitoring data the centre demanded from localities:

> I think there's been a real wasted opportunity in terms of the amount
> of data we feed in regularly to them and I don't see any evidence of it.
> You would have thought they'd have put together an annual publica-
> tion on the work of HAZs. There's been nothing to raise the profile of
> HAZs at the national level and to galvanise that combined force in
> terms of expertise and experience. I think a part of that is that sense of
> nationally not knowing where HAZ is going and it is difficult for them
> to really promote a scheme that might be in danger of having to shut
> down.

Finally, professionals in a number of areas acknowledged that there had
been a *lack of real community involvement* in HAZ activities within their
area. For some, the limited timescales and centrally driven targets had
adversely impacted upon the HAZs' capacity to engage the local public in
their activities. This was considered a significant limitation given that engaging communities was intended to be one of the underpinning principles of
the initiative. This view supports findings outlined in previous chapters; that
HAZs were less successful in their attempts at genuine community involvement in contrast to making more positive progress towards sustainable partnership working between local agencies.

Conclusion

Assessing the impact of any complex initiative is difficult. In the case of
HAZs, the limited lifespan of the initiative and the evaluation, as well as a
lack of good baseline data, made traditional approaches to measuring
change difficult. The influence of a range of local and national factors
restricted the capacity of the zones to realise their original aims and further
complicated any attempts to measure what they have achieved. Given these
limitations, we have attempted to address the issue of impact by drawing on
information from a wide range of sources. In amongst this evidence, some
of it competing, there emerge some important messages about the impact
of Health Action Zones, and perhaps more importantly, how future evaluations should approach this issue.

The review of routinely available health data suggests that, in the short
time in which comparison was possible (1997–2002) there may be some
differences between HAZ and non-HAZ areas. But the differences vary and
there is no clear pattern. In most instances more affluent areas continued to
demonstrate greater improvement than either HAZs or other deprived
areas. In some cases (such as decreases in all cause mortality and CHD

mortality for adults) both first and second wave zones demonstrated greater improvement than other deprived areas. While in other cases (such as mortality rates from suicide) some HAZs (first wave) saw improvements while others (second wave) did not. This variable picture makes it difficult to draw any firm conclusions about the short-term impact of HAZs on the types of health problems and issues recorded in routine statistics.

Amongst those leading HAZs, perceptions of progress and impact were more consistent. Despite what project managers viewed as considerable barriers (primarily in the form of changes at the national level and lack of support from central government) they were united in the view that HAZs had made a positive impact locally. They argued that HAZs had changed ways of working between organisations and implemented a range of useful projects and programmes that benefited local people.

A wider range of stakeholders in eight HAZs identified similar themes. They pointed to a range of individual projects, as well as processes, that they defined as real successes. These ranged from clinical interventions to community-based programmes and specific events or learning tools. Interviewees argued that these activities had made a difference to the lives of individuals and groups living in their area. In addition, many had contributed to realising overall ambitions for the HAZ, particularly in relation to improving services and developing partnerships.

Thus in addressing the question 'What difference does a national initiative such as HAZ make?' the answer is at least twofold. First, it may make some difference at the population level, but this is difficult, if not impossible, to prove in a relatively short period of time. What is more certain is that one can elicit perceptions that it does make a difference at local level, and local actors can provide convincing evidence to support this. This suggests that future evaluations of complex initiatives such as HAZ need to employ a range of research methods and collect data at a range of different levels. Ideally the starting point should be a robust baseline with which to measure changes through time. This is expensive and time-consuming and difficult to collect, but important. Yet it is not enough. More qualitative indicators of success, ideally collected from a range of perspectives, are also needed. It is only through an assessment of both forms of evidence that researchers, practitioners and policy makers can learn more about the different elements of 'what works', and, we hope, use this knowledge to inform future policy.

Chapter 9

Conclusion

Ken Judge and Linda Bauld

Health Action Zones were encouraged to set themselves ambitious goals to improve the health of their communities. Very few of these strategic objectives were accomplished in any very clear or convincing fashion, although as we have shown more modest progress was achieved with individual programmes and projects. Nevertheless, at the most general level there is no escaping the fact that HAZs did not do what they set out to achieve. But it would be wrong to judge them on this basis alone. The truth is much more complex. The nuggets of learning that lie within HAZs have to be mined and cleaned and studied with care. It might appear evasive, but the experience of evaluating HAZs has led us to believe that most 'findings' of real value are context specific and the nature of the question or setting is critical to the learning that can be generated. In this book we have tried to distil some important lessons, but we are acutely conscious that we have only scraped the surface of what there is of value to learn from the HAZ experience. Other colleagues with different perspectives, often as local evaluators, have added to the stock of emerging knowledge (Asthana et al. 2002; Coppel and Dyas 2003; Crawshaw et al. 2003). Inevitably it is the case that different researchers using different lenses for different purposes will arrive at multiple conclusions some of them critical. For our part, however, we want to pay tribute to the fact that many enthusiastic and skilled people worked very hard, often in trying circumstances, to make a success of the HAZ initiative. We often had reason to question in our own minds the appropriateness of this or that course of action as we went about our research activities. But we rarely if ever had reason to doubt the integrity and commitment of the people, communities and organisations that took on the responsibility of promoting sustainable change for disadvantaged groups in the hope that this would eventually lead to a positive transformation of the health prospects of those with the fewest resources.

In the short period of time that Health Action Zones were able to make a direct contribution they engaged in an incredibly diverse range of activities. During the three to four years that most of the zones existed, they sponsored hundreds of workstreams and thousands of projects (Judge et al.

1999). It is astonishingly difficult to capture the complexity of this activity and to aggregate it in any meaningful way to make possible an overall evaluative judgement. As we have outlined, HAZs were not substantial enough and did not survive long enough to make any real impact on conventional indicators of population health or health inequality. But they cannot be dismissed as failures on this basis alone. At their best, HAZs built local capacity and demonstrated change possibilities. They did this in innovative and sustainable ways that will continue to be useful for many years to come. What is important to remember is that the complex myriad of partnerships that constituted Health Action Zones, involving hundreds of organisations and thousands of individuals, means that many different stories can be legitimately told. The result is a mosaic that does not lend itself to easy or brief summary or to unambiguous judgements about success or failure. The simple truth is that we cannot answer the question – what difference did HAZs make – without narrating elaborate stories laden with many qualifications.

A corollary of these observations is that the individual members of the research team have each taken from their evaluation experiences a distinctive set of conclusions based in part on the background knowledge and values that they brought with them. The process of working together and discussing the different elements of the evaluation, of course, means that we hold many views in common. Some of the most important include the need for policy researchers to be as open minded as possible; the value of investigating processes and experiences in their own right and not only as mechanisms that might generate some 'higher level' impact; and the importance of striking a reasonable balance between flexible adaptation in response to changing policy contexts and constancy in pursuit of some stable research themes so as to make effective use of scarce research resources. But there are also many areas where, perfectly reasonably, there is considerable room for differences of opinion about the significance, interpretation and perhaps even the existence of phenomena that some of us regard as important. We do not see this as a problem. We think that there is real value in bringing together these different perspectives, and to do so synergistically, as we have tried to do in this book.

The importance of context

Given the degree of complexity that we, and the Health Action Zones, had to grapple with, a recurrent question in our minds concerns whether or not HAZs were given a fair opportunity to demonstrate what they might have been able to achieve. Their capacity to meet their objectives was significantly and repeatedly affected by a changing context for their work, at local and national level. This context affected both HAZs and our attempts to evaluate their efforts.

From the outset HAZs were encouraged to outbid each other in the scale of their ambitions. Most of them tried to tackle too many seemingly intractable problems simultaneously and they were further hampered by regular attempts by Whitehall to increase and/or to change the focus of their activities. In the heady days of 1998 and 1999 the tidal wave of enthusiasm for the opportunity to engage with the social exclusion agenda meant that local leaders could rise above the day-to-day frustrations of excessive expectations about 'early wins' as they tried to build effective local partnerships. But as the new millennium loomed, the growing preoccupation of health ministers with the restructuring of the NHS posed major problems for Health Action Zones, which were seeking to win the trust of partners, many of whom were suspicious of the medicalisation of health and social problems.

It is no longer fashionable, and probably rightly so, to focus excessive attention on the 'great' men (we use the term advisedly) of history. But it would be wrong not to acknowledge that in many respects Health Action Zones were – in their selection if not entirely in their conception – the creature of Frank Dobson's ambition and orientation. When he was persuaded to resign in 1999 as Secretary of State for Health in a doomed attempt to be elected as the Mayor of London, many of the prospects for Health Action Zones may have gone with him. His successor, Alan Milburn, had a different and more managerial agenda as a result of the growing perception, two or three years into the life of the New Labour government, that key manifesto pledges about the performance of the NHS were in jeopardy. The result was, as Asthana and colleagues (2002) explained:

> The initial emphasis on the need for HAZs to harness local energy, promote innovation and accept risk-taking has given way to an emphasis on the need to achieve national priorities ... funding has been cut and the future of HAZs remains unclear.
>
> (Asthana et al. 2002, p. 785)

The cumulative result of these changes was a crisis in confidence for HAZs. By 2001, many valued leaders became dispirited and moved to other jobs. Those that remained had to deal with the disappointments associated with reduced expectations about funding and the perception that Health Action Zones were yesterday's news. But the very change processes being set in train that seemed to endanger HAZs carried within them the seeds of renewal and opportunity. As things have turned out the Health Action Zone 'badge' will probably be seen to have had a very short shelf life. But HAZs have shown themselves to be capable of making many significant and lasting contributions to the development of local strategic partnerships and primary care trusts. Project managers themselves have been honest enough to acknowledge that progress has been patchy in some areas with perhaps the engagement of front-line staff being seen as the one of the seven founding principles for HAZs where least has been achieved. On the other hand there is considerable optimism that valuable lessons from HAZs are being transferred to other organisations. There is every reason to believe that the spirit of HAZs if not the name will live on.

Key lessons

It would be inappropriate in these final concluding comments to attempt to summarise the detailed contents of earlier chapters. However, a few general points are worth emphasising. These relate to theory-based evaluation; the problem of attribution; the importance of collaboration; planning and targets; whole systems change; measuring outcomes; addressing inequalities and, finally, the challenge of complexity.

One important lesson to emerge from the evaluation reflects both a methodological point and possible guidance to inform future work on strengthening health improvement in practice. We began with high expectations about the use of theory-based evaluation in general and theories of change in particular. For a whole series of reasons, which we have discussed elsewhere (Judge and Bauld 2001; Judge and Mackenzie 2002; Sullivan et al. 2002; Barnes et al. 2003b), this did not materialise in the way that we had originally hoped. Our expectation that local actors could be persuaded to articulate and adhere to sophisticated strategies for change contained a large element of wishful thinking. There is also a real sense in which the approach assumes too much of a linear view of the world, which is at odds with the continuous process of interaction and adjustment to changing circumstances experienced by local actors. But this does not mean that the Theory of Change approach is without value. It can and does help local planning. It could perhaps do so to an even greater extent than we have observed. Our experience suggests it is easier for practitioners to accommodate it at programme or project level, whereas attempting to create a Theory of Change at the strategic level is much more demanding. But whatever level the approach is used for it does have enormous potential for promoting good planning and asking important questions about issues of evaluability: what are the prospects of generating robust learning from an initiative. In addition, the approach might have a different and possibly equally valuable contribution to building the evidence base for effective social change. If time and effort can be put into working with local actors retrospectively, to create theories of what and why things *happened*, in addition to prospectively eliciting notions of the ways in which things *might change*, then it might be possible to realise Weiss's (1995b) claim that there is nothing as practical as good theory in a rich variety of ways.

Another important general point that we emphasise in a number of ways is that so many things were happening in HAZ areas simultaneously that it is often very difficult to know which initiative or organisation contributed precisely what to any particular activity. A rich and varied mix of local actors and organisations took advantage of a wide range of opportunities to further their shared social goals and aspirations. Thus, *attributing* who did what and when to what effect was made even more difficult, something which local stakeholders themselves acknowledged in their own assessment of HAZ impact (Sullivan et al. 2004). HAZs were part of a rich and changing kaleidoscope of local activity and it is precisely such engagement that is an important part of their success, but the varied nature of their complex interrelationships with multiple initiatives militates against a very precise attribution of what specifically contributed to what. Of course, this does not mean that issues of attribution can be neglected. Indeed one of the claims made for theory-based approaches is that the prospective specification of plausible change pathways that can be measured and monitored makes a very valuable contribution to the learning process. But much depends on the quality both of the theory and the monitoring mechanisms and in practice these often prove to be inadequate, in part because of the relatively limited and marginal role that is afforded to the monitoring function, and also because of the genuine difficulties that exist in relation to delineating evidence of outcomes in complex policy areas.

One of the most important points arising from observing the complex diversity of local activity is perhaps one of the most obvious. Building effective local partnerships is not possible without taking very seriously the strengthening of both individual and organisational capacity. But other preconditions are also essential. Sullivan et al. (2002) show that collaboration works best where there is at least a partial coincidence of interests and values, where there is mutual respect for plurality and difference in terms of purpose and priority, where there is a degree of stability and sufficient time to build trust and ownership of agendas and where resources of many kinds are made available to lubricate and glue together the diverse activities of individuals, communities and organisations. Particular attention also needs to be paid to the roles that are identified for 'the public' in these programmes and the kinds of support that may be needed for these roles to be realised in contexts where long standing power relationships will act to delimit the possibilities for change.

Another key message that cuts across much of the evaluation, and which we have already alluded to, is that for entities such as Health Action Zones to make an impact it is essential that they recognise the importance of clarity of purpose and planning. Yet, throughout the lifetime of HAZs this was problematic. One of the main conclusions in our very first report to the DH in 1999 echoed this theme:

> Health Action Zones are required to produce explicit targets. But there
> has been quite a lot of confusion about what constitutes an appropriate
> target. While to varying degrees all of the implementation plans are

strong on identifying problems, articulating long-term objectives and specifying routinely available indicators for monitoring progress, they are much less good at filling the gap between problems and goals. Only in very rare cases is it possible to identify a clear and logical pathway which links problems, strategies for intervention, milestones or targets with associated time-scales and longer-term outcomes. Most importantly, and most frequently, specific 'targets' were highlighted without any accompanying explanation of the mechanisms intended to achieve them. This omission is key. It breaks the critical link between the problems that HAZs are there to address and the ambitious goals that they rightly wish to set for themselves.

(Judge et al. 1999, pp. 30–1)

In his second report, *Securing Good Health for the Whole Population* (2004), Derek Wanless draws attention to some of the problems inherent in target-setting. He argues that:

they have not always met the requirements of stretching ambition and realism. The philosophies behind them have been inconsistent. So, the smoking targets set in 1998 could be considered unambitious while the obesity targets (1992) and the physical activity target (2002) seem highly aspirational. In none of these cases does the target setting process encourage a belief that resource management to achieve improvement will be optimal.

(Wanless 2004, p. 6)

Another key finding from Chapter 6 that is based on a considerable process of discussion and observation in Health Action Zones, is that it is essential that three key processes must be fostered if sustainable processes of whole systems change are to be put in place.

* an understanding of the cycle of change and its concomitant barriers/drivers at a national and local level
* an understanding of context (for example, in terms of local needs, organisational structures and capacity for collaboration) as the starting point for any complex, community initiative
* a commitment to building evaluation and mainstreaming structures into the initial development of strategy.

An explicit recognition of the importance of these points has to be part of the process of making and monitoring policy at a national level as well as the practical means of implementation at a more local level.

It is also important that a more sophisticated approach is taken to the measurement of outcomes in relation to the evaluation of complex community-based initiatives such as HAZs. Fortunately, there are growing signs that this message has been received in Whitehall. For example, a 'taking stock and looking to the future' document produced by the Social Exclusion Unit (2004) acknowledges that new approaches need to be developed to produce theoretically plausible intermediate indicators of whether or not progress is being made in relation to the primary outcomes of interest.

> The success of many current policies is measured by 'hard' or quantifiable outcomes, such as movement into work or gaining a qualification, which are very important for us to monitor and measure success by. 'Soft' outcomes, such as increased personal confidence, could be seen as being important to some people, particularly those who are most vulnerable. These may be necessary first steps in achieving longer-term outcomes such as moving into work or training in the future. These intermediate outcomes are not currently measured or routinely captured in targets and can be very difficult to measure. Where these soft outcomes can be clearly related to the longer-term achievement of hard outcomes, mechanisms for capturing this information would be valuable.
>
> (Social Exclusion Unit 2004, p. 23)

Benzeval's findings in Chapter 7 also shed light on the practical difficulties associated with trying to address inequalities in health. While there has always been evident enthusiasm for the importance of tackling health inequalities this has been tempered with realism. Virtually without exception, everyone that members of the research team ever spoke to during the course of the national evaluation articulated concerns about the limited resources and time available to HAZs to make any realistic impact on inequality. As a result the primary ambition of HAZs was to make sure that equity issues were firmly placed on the agendas of a wide range of agencies, and that local capacity was built to maintain sustained efforts to reduce inequalities. It is perhaps in this area that HAZs have had most success. But it is clear that much remains to be done even in terms of preparatory work. Benzeval highlights five areas where there is particular need to make more progress in building capacity.

* defining the nature of the problem
* widening understanding of causes
* strengthening the evidence base
* making equity activity more part of the mainstream
* finding imaginative ways of measuring progress in the medium term.

The final substantive point to make is that in many important ways HAZs were victims of the complexity that they set out to address. The biggest obstacle of all, to which no clear solution has been found by practitioners or researchers, is what Pawson (2003, p. 472) describes as 'the utter and appalling intricacy of social interventions'. What is now badly needed is a new body of theory about what it is reasonable to expect community-based social programmes to deliver in the face of the bewildering scale of the complexities that they face. A central aspect of this general point is that the initiatives and interventions that are the subject of evaluation have to be organised and implemented in a way that enables them to address answerable questions.

For example, our experience of evaluating Health Action Zones strongly reinforces the importance of some of the comments made by Derek Wanless (2004). He points out that although 'there is often evidence on the scientific justification for action and for some specific interventions, there is generally little evidence about the cost-effectiveness of public health and preventative policies or their practical implementation' (Wanless 2004, p. 5). One of the consequences of this central weakness in the evidence base for promoting population health and reducing health inequalities is that policy initiatives are often not thought through with sufficient care at the time when they are conceived and announced:

> This has led to the introduction of a very wide range of initiatives, often with unclear objectives and little quantification of outcomes and it has meant it is difficult to sustain support for initiatives, even those which are successful. It is evident that a great deal more discipline is needed to ensure problems are clearly identified and tackled, that the multiple solutions frequently needed are sensibly co-ordinated and that lessons are learnt which feed back directly into policy.
>
> (Wanless 2004, p. 5)

Nevertheless, Wanless goes on to emphasise the huge potential value that would be realised by strengthening the evaluation of many existing and new programmes. But in order to take full advantage of following the injunction that 'every opportunity to generate evidence from current policy and practice needs to be realized', there are important lessons to be learnt about the design and implementation of substantial community-based social interventions such as HAZs.

Implications for policy research

With the benefit of hindsight it is relatively easy but perhaps not helpful to suggest that both the design of the HAZ initiative and the commissioning of its evaluation could have been undertaken with greater care and considerably more realism. Yet the experience of evaluating HAZs does suggest that some things could have been done differently, and that some decisions should have been more carefully considered, particularly in light of the experience of other initiatives and other evaluations that had gone before. More generally, consideration needs to be given to the design of complex initiatives and the extent to which they lend themselves to evaluation. We can also comment on our experience of conducting the evaluation and can reflect on how things might have been done differently. Finally, it is worth reflecting on practical lessons for evaluating complex interventions.

Programme design and 'evaluability'

Health Action Zones were born in the heady of days of the summer of 1997 after an historic election victory. In many ways anything seemed possible for a New Labour government desperate to demonstrate its capacity to make things work and quickly. Moreover, they were encouraged by many of the people and organisations working with and for the most socially excluded and disadvantaged groups. There was an enormous appetite and enthusiasm for swift action to tackle the modern version of Beveridge's 'five giants' of want, disease, ignorance, squalor and idleness (Timmins 1995). But with the benefit of hindsight, more than seven years on, it does seem that the tide of enthusiasm for change outran the capacity to deliver it. Too many hugely ambitious and aspirational targets were promulgated. The pressure to produce 'early wins' became debilitating, and a sense of disillusionment began to set in.

The notion that an injection of relatively modest resources accompanied by guidance – more evangelical than practical – from Whitehall might result in the speedy resolution of major social problems, that had proved largely intractable for generations, would not find many advocates at the present time even in government (Social Exclusion Unit 2004). From very early on, HAZs were put under considerable pressure to demonstrate that they were 'making a difference' within a relatively short time period. Yet, as Alcock (2004, p. 95), writing about area-based initiatives, has put it: 'early hits are not always evidence of accurate shooting'. There are clearly lessons to be learnt about the design and implementation of substantial community-based social interventions such as HAZs. There is a need to think more carefully about the focus of such initiatives, their objectives, their timescales, the support that they need both locally and nationally and the space and trust and time that is required to make any kind of sustainable change possible.

In particular, it is absolutely essential to make greater efforts to maximise genuine learning opportunities from all of the investments that are being made to improve health and reduce inequalities. Wanless makes the same point.

> Given the limited evidence base for public health, every opportunity to generate evidence from current policy and practice needs to be realized.

Much of public health policy and practice currently being implemented has not been rigorously evaluated to assess its effectiveness. Many in the research community highlight the potential of public health programmes for use as natural experiments, where evaluation should be an explicit component of the implementation of new interventions, programmes and policies, and so could inform the evidence base for public health.

(Wanless 2004, pp. 114–15).

But he would have been well advised to say more about the fundamental issue of evaluability. One of the major problems is that many initiatives are not designed and implemented in ways that lend themselves to learning, and many evaluations are commissioned in ways that fail to acknowledge sufficiently the many practical constraints associated with policy research. Commissioning studies of initiatives with poorly specified objectives in the interests of generating 'evidence' is often a waste of scarce research resources. As other commentators have noted, researchers attempting to evaluate such initiatives often spend a great deal of time and effort supporting the development and implementation of the programme (Evans et al. 2001). They may come up with complex and often contradictory findings that policy makers find difficult to digest, and therefore ignore, rather than using them to inform future decisions. Part of the problem is one of expectation. Too many users of policy research still expect clear answers about impact when a more realistic product of evaluations is that they contribute to a process of enlightenment about highly complex processes that are interpreted by different actors in multiple ways.

Our experience

As far as our own experience of being commissioned to undertake the evaluation of HAZs is concerned, it seems to us with the benefit of hindsight that there was a much clearer sense within the Department of Health in 1997/98 that HAZs *had* to be evaluated than *why* or *how*. That is perhaps why the commissioning process took so long to complete, the resources available to conduct any evaluation of potential impact were so small, and the expectations of policy customers seemed ever changing. We tried on numerous occasions, and with some success, to insist on a degree of realism about the focus of the evaluation, but throughout its life some of us felt like we were chasing elusive shadows as we continually tried to adapt to the needs of sponsors hungry for evidence. This is not because we were working with people who lacked integrity, far from it. Everyone that we worked with tried to be supportive. However, many of the civil servants we had dealings with had several competing pressures on their time in what was often a bewilderingly fast-moving policy world.

At least in part, of course, we were guilty of a degree of naivety as a team in thinking that we might contribute more than we could. In the early stages we invested perhaps too much effort in animating and promoting the initiative at the expense of clear thinking about some aspects of feasible research design. But whatever our limitations, in these or other respects, we certainly began to have growing concerns about the pressure to generate and use learning at too early a stage in the cycle of data collection, analysis and reflection. It seems to us that there is a real possibility that the mantra of evidence-based policy-making and practice will actually constrain the capacity to produce genuinely valuable learning about what works for whom in what circumstances. Simply documenting activity, which is frequently demanded and regularly served up, is not evidence of good practice and the growing tendency to pretend that it does yields little more than glossy propaganda. But once again our experience reminds us that different audiences or customers for policy research need different products. More dialogue with key stakeholders about what a research team can produce, as well as what is not possible, and explicit agreements about what are the key priorities, are important and virtually continuous parts of the research process. Without this investment of time and understanding there is enormous potential for policy users and research producers to continue to disappoint each other.

The kinds of enlightenment evaluation about key processes, such as community participation reported in this book, can help to meet the needs of new organisations such as PCTs that have limited knowledge about how best to respond to the latest set of priorities from Whitehall. But the richness, and what is often the context-specific nature, of such research can make the process of dissemination and digestion a difficult one. Furthermore, even the best examples of such research cannot answer all of the questions that policymakers and practitioners want guidance about. The problem then is that the universally voracious appetite for intelligence encourages the production of simple descriptions of activity without adequate discussion of the strengths and weaknesses of what is being presented. When this point is reached it would be a much more valuable contribution to the public good to admit more often that we do not have clear answers to what may seem pressing problems.

It is often argued that the really significant contributions to strengthening the evidence base to tackle health inequalities, for example, will come from well-designed studies that set out to answer clearly defined questions. As we have already implied, this will not be possible unless the interventions to be evaluated are themselves designed with more rigour than is commonplace. Nevertheless, it seems unlikely that the frequent dash to intervene in response to the latest crisis or problem to reach the political hit list will not continue to be part of the political landscape in modern democracies. There is a real danger in these circumstances, especially when the imperative to intervene quickly is combined with unrealistic expectations about the speed with which research findings can be generated, that valuable learning opportunities will be missed. The challenge when evaluation opportunities arise in the wake of such interventions is to negotiate the best possible research approach that acknowledges *inter alia* that incontrovertible measures of impact are not the only the useful products that can be generated. The value of shining a light on complex processes in reflective and scholarly ways should not be underestimated even if it falls some way short of what is ideally required.

It is a matter of some regret that Health Action Zones are perhaps best perceived as an example of the 'hit and run' mentality of early New Labour enthusiasm. This is not so much a matter of blame or competence but rather one of circumstance. Nevertheless, given the resources that the evaluation consumed it is worth asking what further contribution it might make. In the late 1990s and early 2000s the DH and other government departments commissioned a number of evaluations of complex policy initiatives such as total purchasing pilots and HAZs and numerous others (Stewart et al. 1999; Evans et al. 2001; Russell 2001; Barnes, J. et al. 2003). There would be great merit in commissioning a short critical review of the experience of, and value associated with, these research studies. Each of these studies adopted a slightly different approach, used a different combination of research methods, and involved researchers from different disciplinary backgrounds. Yet many seem to have come up with similar conclusions about some of the challenges and pitfalls of attempting to evaluate complex policy initiatives, particularly those that are area based. Several offer practical suggestions about how studies can adapt to, for example a changing policy context or political agenda, and how to resolve tensions between supporting and evaluating an initiative. A review of these studies could be of real value, with a view to establishing clearer guidance for future evaluations. Of course, it is extremely unlikely that such a review would invent a new methodology for conducting evaluations, but a distillation of experience in a number of policy areas would provide useful guidance for commissioners of such studies in the future.

Thus, in our view, it would be wrong to zero in on HAZs or any other recent initiative in isolation. Health Action Zones were part of a large body of area-based initiatives and any real learning will come from reviewing some or all of them in combination. In fact, what is also needed is a critical review of the design, implementation and achievements of the many complex social interventions introduced in the United Kingdom in recent years. In the absence of such a review we conclude with some practical lessons for evaluating complex interventions. Inspired by a leading practitioner in the field of theory-based evaluation; we have borrowed the framework of Pawson's (2003, p. 486) 'six tips for getting intimate with intricacy', but the suggestions we make are based on our own experiences and in some important respects differ from his.

'Getting intimate with intricacy'

The more important and challenging is the problem to be faced and the more ambitious is the intervention that is proposed to deal with it the greater the degree of complexity that has to be faced by both implementers and evaluators. The precise form of that complexity differs from one initiative to another but there are a number of common strands.

The basic ingredients of complexity, however, are always there. There is always an implementation chain, running through policy makers, practitioners and subjects. There is always negotiation about the precise delivery of the intervention. There is always borrowing of programme theory from parallel initiatives. There is always the historical legacy of previous reforms. And evaluators are always left with the same question – complexity is inescapable, what can be done in the face of it (Pawson 2003, pp. 485–6)?

There is no single or easy answer, but as experience of undertaking evaluations of complex initiatives grows and is shared a growing number of practical suggestions are emerging. We use Pawson's (2003, p. 486) headings for his 'tips on getting to grips with intricacy' to outline our own recommendations.

Stare it in the face

Logic models and conceptual maps of what an initiative is trying to do are not easy to produce but they are extremely valuable. The process of encouraging key stakeholders to articulate their thoughts and assumptions about key parts of the postulated change process, even when significant gaps remain, is essential. But this should not be done to exhaustion. Consensus though desirable is not essential and too much emphasis on seeking a single theory of change may be more harmful than helpful. The key thing is to produce a recognisable narrative picture that is meaningful and recognisable to the key actors involved. We cannot pretend that this process is an easy one. But skilled and experienced researchers can make a very useful contribution (Mackenzie and Blamey 2005).

Concentrate your fire

The principal purpose of the map for the evaluator is to facilitate decisions about where the major research effort should be concentrated. It is extremely unlikely that it will ever be possible in practice to investigate every interesting aspect of complex initiatives. Choices have to be made about where and how to deploy scarce research resources. This selection has to be negotiated with research commissioners and local implementers but the potentially successful evaluator must stand their ground and persuade everyone concerned that only so much can be examined properly and that the emphasis must be on what are regarded as the critical change mechanisms.

It is perhaps worth emphasising that in this respect we have in mind the possibility of focussing attention at a rather higher level of generality than that suggested by Pawson (2003), but the actual choice in any particular evaluation situation will always have to be at least in part a function of content, resources and theory.

Go back to the future

It is important not to be constrained by the initiative itself. Really good policy research has to be dynamic and well connected with developments in other areas. The greatest impact will be generated by linking even half-formed impressions from specific research studies with the main currents of learning that are continually emerging in other geographic and policy settings. Locating specific programmes in the wider societal developments of which they are inevitably a part and making effective linkages between different aspects of learning will increase the probability that researchers can make effective contributions to future policy and practice development. Scholarship is as much an integral part of good quality policy research as in any other field of inquiry.

Stand on others' shoulders

A crucial aspect of making effective linkages is to be humble and scholarly. Even though an initiative might look like a significant innovation and its ambition and scope appears new and exciting it will have many precursors. Many of its building blocks will have been evaluated in some form before. Policy research is not a good setting for reinventing wheels. Systematic reviews of existing knowledge can help with the process of concentrating scarce evaluation effort so that it is used to maximum effect.

Criss and cross

In making the selection of which mechanisms to choose for close scrutiny it is useful to remember the value to be obtained by combining horizontal and vertical perspectives about different aspects of an intervention. No matter how interesting a single project in a single place might look, much more learning stands to be obtained by including substantial comparative elements in the selected research design. If one takes community participation as an example, there is much to be learnt from the existing research literature and from tracing through specific examples in particular contexts, but considerable research value can be added by criss-crossing between the horizontal investigation of particular approaches to participation with all of their individual nuances and a vertical comparison of how similar elements of the mechanism of interest work in different contexts.

Remember your job

Complex community-based initiatives are just that. They do not lend themselves to simple calculations of good or bad, right or wrong, successful or not. The job of the policy researcher is to illuminate the processes of change and experience that they observe. In doing so one can contribute to a collective process of 'enlightenment' about complex change processes in modern social welfare systems. The policy researcher should, therefore, use every evaluation opportunity to shine the light on some important aspect of the process either of their own choosing or that can best be negotiated with programme sponsors and research commissioners. The ethical obligation of the policy researcher is to make a contribution – albeit a modest one – to the social process of understanding and promoting change. It is not to award or withhold a seal of approval to this or that 'flavour of the moment' initiative that might have provided the pretext for a new investigative opportunity.

A corollary of these final thoughts is that any lasting value associated with the evaluation of Health Action Zones is most likely to be that it will contribute to a stock of knowledge that future policy researchers can draw upon. Despite the difficulties and frustration that we have encountered, we continue to believe that there is much of value to learn from the experience of HAZs, especially at a time when concerted efforts to improve the equitable distribution of population health are assuming growing importance in an increasing number of societies.

References

6 P (1997) *Holistic Government*. London: DEMOS.

6 P., Leat, D., Seltzer, K. and Stoker, G. (1999) *Governing in the Round: Strategies for Holistic Government*. London: DEMOS.

Abbott, S., Florin, D., Fulop, N. and Gillam, S. (2001) *Primary Care Groups and Trusts: Improving Health*. London: King's Fund.

Acheson, D. (1998) *Independent Inquiry into Inequalities into Health*. London: The Stationery Office.

Adams, C., Bauld, L. and Judge, K. (2000) *Leading the Way: Smoking Cessation Services in Health Action Zones*. Glasgow: Health Promotion Policy Unit, University of Glasgow. Online. Available http://www.haznet.org.uk/.

Alcock, A. (2004) 'Participation or pathology: contradictory tensions in area-based policy', *Social Policy and Society*, 3: 87–96.

Anand, S. (2002) 'The concern for equity in health', *Journal of Epidemiology and Community Health*, 56: 485–7.

Annandale, E. and Hunt, K. (eds.) (2000) *Gender Inequalities in Health*. Buckingham: Open University Press.

Ashton, J. and Seymour, H. (1988) *The New Public Health: the Liverpool Experience*. Milton Keynes: Open University Press.

Asthana, S., Richardson, S. and Halliday, J. (2002) 'Partnership working in public policy provision: a framework for evaluation', *Social Policy and Administration*, 36: 780–95.

Atkinson, A.B., Rainwater, L. and Smeeding, T.M. (1995) *Income Distribution in OECD Countries*, Social policy studies no. 18. Paris: OECD.

Audit Commission (1989) *Urban Regeneration and Economic Development: The Local Government Dimension*. London: HMSO.

Audit Commission (2002) *Neighbourhood Renewal*. London: Audit Commission.

Barnekov, T., Boyle, R., and Rich, D. (1990) *Privatism and Urban Policy in Britain and the USA*. Oxford: Oxford University Press.

Barnes, J., Broomfield, J., Frost, M., Harper, G., McLeod, A., Knowles, J. and Leyland, A. (2003) *Characteristics of Sure Start Local Programme Areas*, Rounds 1–4, National Evaluation of Sure Start. London: DfES Publications. Online. Available http:www.surestart.gov.uk.

Barnes, M. (1997a) *Care, Communities and Citizens*. London: Addison Wesley Longman.

Barnes, M. (1997b) *The People's Health Service?* Birmingham: HSMC, University of Birmingham/NHS Confederation.

Barnes, M. (1999a) 'Users as citizens: collective action and the local governance of welfare', *Social Policy and Administration*, 33: 73–90.

Barnes, M. (1999b) *From Paternalism to Partnership: Changing Relationships in Health and Health Services*, no. 10 in the Policy Futures for UK Health Technical Series. Cambridge: The Nuffield Trust/University of Cambridge Judge Institute of Management Studies.

Barnes, M. (2002) 'Dialogue between older people and public officials: UK experiences', in *Grey Power? Volume 1: Political Power and Influence*, Les Cahiers de la FIAPA. Action Research on Ageing, 2: 166–82.

Barnes, M. and Bennet, G. (1998) 'Frail bodies, courageous voices: older people influencing community care', *Health and Social Care in the Community*, 6: 102–11.

Barnes, M. and Bowl, R. (2001) *Taking Over the Asylum: Empowerment and Mental Health*. Basingstoke: Palgrave.

Barnes, M. and Prior, D. (1995) 'Spoilt for choice? How consumerism can disempower public service users', *Public Money and Management*, 15: 53–8.

Barnes, M. and Prior, D. (1996) 'From private choice to public trust: a new social basis for welfare', *Public Money and Management*, 16: 51–8.

Barnes, M. and Prior, D. (1998) 'Trust and the competence of the welfare consumer', in A. Coulson (ed.) *Trust and Contracts: Relationships in Local Government, Health and Public Services*. Bristol: Policy Press.

Barnes, M. and Prior, D. (2000) *Private Lives as Public Policy*. Birmingham: Venture Press.

Barnes, M., Knops, A., Newman, J. and Sullivan, H. (2002) *Power, Participation and Political Renewal*, final report to ESRC of a research project undertaken in the Democracy and Participation Research programme. Birmingham: University of Birmingham.

Barnes, M., Matka, E. and Sullivan, H. (2001) Context, Strategy and Capacity: Interim findings from the strategic level analysis. Building Capacity for Collaboration, National Evaluation of Health Action Zones, University of Birmingham.

Barnes, M., Matka, E. and Sullivan, H. (2003a) 'Evidence, understanding and complexity: evaluation in non-linear systems', *Evaluation*, 9: 263–82.

Barnes, M., Sullivan, H. and Matka, E. (2003b) *The Development of Collaborative Capacity in Health Action Zones*, final report from the national evaluation. Birmingham: University of Birmingham.

Barnes, M., Knops, A., Newman, J. and Sullivan, H. (2004a) 'The micro-politics of deliberation: case studies in public participation', *Contemporary Politics*, 10: 93–110.

Barnes, M., Sullivan, H. and Matka, E. (2004b) *Building Capacity for Collaboration*, final report of the HAZ national evaluation. Birmingham: University of Birmingham.

Barnes, M., Sullivan, H., Knops, A., and Newman, J. (2004) 'Power, participation and political renewal: a study of public participation in two English cities'. IDS Bulletin, University of Sussex, vol. 12, no. 2, pp. 58–66.

Bauld, L., Coleman, T., Adams, C., Pound, E. and Ferguson, J. (2005) 'Delivering the English Smoking Treatment Services', *Addiction*, 100 suppl 2: 19–27.

Bauld, L., Judge, K., Lawson, L., Mackenzie, M., Mackinnon, J. and Truman, J. (2001a) *Health Action Zones in Transition: Progress in 2000.* Glasgow: Health Promotion Policy Unit, University of Glasgow. Online. Available http://www.haznet.org.uk.

Bauld, L., Mackinnon, J. and Judge, K. (2001b) *Community Health Initiatives: Recent Policy Developments and The Emerging Evidence-Base.* London: Neighbourhood Renewal Unit, Office of the Deputy Prime Minister. Online. Available http://www.neighbourhood.gov/research.asp.

Bauld, L., Butler, R., Hay, G., Judge, K. and McKeganey, N. (2002) *Drug Prevention for Vulnerable Young People: Mapping Pump-priming Projects in Health Action Zones.* Glasgow: Health Promotion Policy Unit, University of Glasgow.

Bauld, L., Chesterman, J., Judge, K., Pound, E. and Coleman, T. (2003) 'Impact of UK National Health Service smoking cessation services: variations in outcomes in England', *Tobacco Control,* 12: 296–301.

Beer, M., Eisenstat, R. and Spector, B. (1990) *The Critical Path Approach to Corporate Renewal.* Boston, MA: Harvard Business School Press.

Benyon, J. and Edwards, A. (1999) 'Community governance of crime control', in G. Stoker (ed.) *The New Management of British Local Governance.* London: Macmillan.

Benzeval, M. (1997) 'Health', in A. Walker and C. Walker (eds) *Britain Divided: the Growth of Social Exclusion in the 1980s and 1990s.* London: CPAG, pp. 153–69.

Benzeval, M. (1999) 'Health inequalities: public policy action', in S. Griffiths and D. Hunter (eds) *Perspectives in Public Health.* Oxford: Radcliffe Medical Press, pp. 34–46.

Benzeval, M. (2002) 'England', in J. Mackenbach and M. Bakker (eds) *Reducing Inequalities in Health: A European Perspective.* London: Routledge.

Benzeval, M. (2003a) *The Final Report of the Tackling Inequalities in Health Module: The National Evaluation of Health Action Zones,* a report to the Department of Health. London: Department of Geography, Queen Mary, University of London. Online. Available http://www.geog.qmw.ac.uk/staff/pdf/finalreport1.pdf.

Benzeval, M. (2003b) *Tackling Inequalities in Health Module: The Final Report to East London and the City Health Action Zone.* London: Department of Geography, Queen Mary, University of London. Online. Available at http://www.geog.qmul.ac.uk/health/publications.

Benzeval, M. (2003c) *Tackling Inequalities in Health Module: The Final Report to North Staffordshire Health Action Zone.* London: Department of Geography, Queen Mary, University of London. Online. Available at http://www.geog.qmul.ac.uk/health/publications.

Benzeval, M. (2003d) *Tackling Inequalities in Health Module: The Final Report to Sheffield Health Action Zone.* London: Department of Geography, Queen Mary, University of London. Online. Available at http://www.geog.qmul.ac.uk/health/publications.

Benzeval, M. and Meth, F. (2002a) *Health Inequalities: A Priority at a Crossroads, Final Report to the Department of Health.* London: Department of Geography, Queen Mary, University of London. Online. Available http://www.geog.qmw.ac.uk/health/publications.

Benzeval, M. and Meth, F. (2002b) 'Innovation', in L. Bauld and K. Judge (eds) *Learning from Health Action Zones.* Chichester: Aeneas.

Benzeval, M., Judge, K. and Smaje, C. (1995a) 'Beyond class, race and ethnicity: deprivation and health in Britain', *Health Services Research*, 30: 163–77.

Benzeval, M., Judge, K. and Whitehead, M. (1995b) *Tackling Inequalities in Health: An Agenda for Action*. London: King's Fund.

Benzeval, M., Taylor, J. and Judge, K. (2000) 'Evidence on the relationship between low income and poor health: is the government doing enough?', *Fiscal Studies*, 21: 375–99.

Beresford, P. and Croft, S. (1993) *Citizen Involvement: A Practical Guide for Change*. London: Macmillan.

Berghman, J. (1995) 'Social exclusion in Europe: policy context and analytical framework', in G. Room (ed.) *Beyond the Threshold: The Measurement and Analysis of Social Exclusion*. Bristol: Policy Press.

Bertalanffy, L. von (1952) *General Systems Theory*. New York: Wiley.

Black, N. (2001) 'Evidence based policy: proceed with care', *BMJ*, 323: 275–8.

Blamey, A. (2001) *Have a Heart Paisley: Report on the Theories of Change Development*. Glasgow: Health Promotion Policy Unit, University of Glasgow.

Blamey, A., Judge, K. and Mackenzie, M. (2002) 'Theory-based evaluation of complex community based health initiatives', a paper presented at the Tackling Health Inequalities: Turning Policy into Practice HDA Seminar. London: Health Development Agency.

Bradford, M. and Robson, B. (1995) 'An evaluation of urban policy', in R. Hambleton and H. Thomas (eds) *Urban Policy Evaluation: Challenge and Change*. London: Paul Chapman

Braveman, P. and Gruskin, S. (2003) 'Defining equity in health', *Journal of Epidemiology and Community Health*, 57: 254–8.

Bryson, J. (1988) 'Strategic planning – big wins and small wins', *Public Money and Management*, 8: 11–15.

Campbell, D. and Stanley, J. (1966) *Experimental and Quasi-experimental Designs for Research*. Chicago: Rand McNally.

Campbell, J. and Oliver, M. (1996) *Disability Politics: Understanding our Past, Changing our Future*. London: Routledge.

Campbell, M., Fitzpatrick, R., Haines, A., Kinmonth, A., Sandercock, P., Spiegelhalter, D. and Tyrer, P. (2000) 'Framework for design and evaluation of complex interventions to improve health', *British Medical Journal*, 321: 694–6.

Carlisle, S. (2001) 'Inequalities in health: contested explanations, shifting discourses and ambiguous policies', *Critical Public Health*, 11: 2001.

Castle, P. and Jacobson, B. (1988) *The Health of our Regions: an Analysis of the Strategies and Policies of Regional Health Authorities for Promoting Health and Preventing Disease. A Report for the Health Education Council*. Birmingham: NHS Regions Health Promotion Group.

Cattell, V. (2001) 'Poor people, poor places and poor health: the mediating role of social networks and social capital', *Social Science and Medicine*, 52: 1501–16.

Challis, L., Fuller, S., Henwood, M., Klein, R., Plowden, W., Webb, A., Whittingham, P. and Wistow, G. (1988) *Joint Approaches to Social Policy*. Cambridge: Cambridge University Press.

Chapman, J. (2002) *System Failure: Why Governments must Learn to Think Differently*. London: Demos.

Checkland, P. (1981) *Systems Thinking; Systems Practice*. New York: Wiley.

Checkland, P. and Scholes, J. (1990) *Soft Systems Methodology in Action*. Chichester: Wiley.

Chen, H.T. (1990) *Theory-Driven Evaluation*. London: Sage.

Church, K. (1996) 'Beyond "Bad Manners": the power relations of "Consumer Participation" in Ontario's Community Mental Health System', *Canadian Journal of Community Mental Health*, 15: 27–44.

Clarence, E. and Painter, C. (1998) 'Public services under New Labour: collaborative discourses and local networking', *Public Policy and Administration*, 13: 8–22.

Clarke, J. and Newman, J. (1997) *The Managerial State: Power, Politics and Ideology in the Remaking of Social Welfare*. London: Sage.

Clarke, M. and Stewart, J. (1997) *Handling the Wicked Issues: A Challenge for Government*. Birmingham: INLOGOV, University of Birmingham.

Cockburn, C. (1977) *The Local State*. London: Pluto.

Coleman, T., Pound, E., Adams, C., Bauld, L., Ferguson, J. and Cheater, F. (2005) 'Implementing a national treatment service for dependent smokers: initial challenges and solutions', *Addiction*, 100 suppl 2: 12–18.

Connell, J. and Kubisch, A. (1998) 'Applying a theory of change approach to the evaluation of comprehensive community initiatives: progress, prospects and problems', in K. Fulbright-Anderson, A. Kubisch and J. Connell (eds) *New Approaches to Evaluating Community Initiatives: Volume 2, Theory, Measurement, and Analysis*, Washington, DC: The Aspen Institute.

Connell, J.P., Kubisch, A.C., Schorr, L.B. and Weiss, C.H. (1995) *New Approaches to Evaluating Community Initiatives. Volume 1: Concepts, Methods and Contexts*. Washington, DC: The Aspen Institute.

Cook, D. (2002) 'Consultation, for a change? Engaging users and communities in the policy process', *Social Policy and Administration*, 36: 516–31.

Cooper, H., Arber, S. and Ginn, J. (1999) *The Influence of Social Support and Social Capital on Health: A Review and Analysis of British Data*. London: Health Education Authority.

Coppel, D. and Dyas, J. (2003) 'Strengthening the links between health action zone evaluation and primary care research', *Primary Health Care Research and Development*, 4: 39–47.

Crawshaw, P., Bunton, R. and Gillen, K. (2002) 'Modernisation and Health Action Zones: the search for coherence', in L. Bauld and K. Judge (eds) *Learning from Health Action Zones*. Chichester: Aeneas.

Crawshaw, P., Bunton, R., and Gillen, K. (2003) 'Health Action Zones and the problem of community', *Health and Social Care in the Community*, 11: 36–44.

Cropper, S. (1996) 'Collaborative working and the issue of sustainability', in C. Huxham (ed.) *Creating Collaborative Advantage*. London: Sage.

Curtis, S. (2004) *Health and Inequality: Geographical Perspectives*. London: Sage.

Curtis, S., Cave, B. and Coutts, A. (2002) 'Is urban regeneration good for health? Perceptions and theories of the health impacts of urban change', *Environment and Planning C*, 20: 517–34.

Dahler-Larsen, P. (2001) 'From programme theory to constructivism: on tragic, magic and competing programmes', *Evaluation*, 7: 331–49.

Davey Smith, G., Ebrahim, S. and Frankel, S. (2001) 'How policy informs the evidence: evidence-based thinking can lead to debased policy making', *British Medical Journal*, 322: 184–5.

Davey Smith, G., Dorling, D., Mitchell, R. and Shaw, M. (2002) 'Health inequalities in Britain: continuing increases up to the end of the 20th century', *Journal of Epidemiology and Community Health*, 56: 434–5.

Davies, H., Nutley, S. and Smith, P. (1999) 'Editorial: What Works? The role of evidence in public sector policy and practice', *Public Money and Management*, 19: 3–4.

Davies, H., Nutley, S. and Smith, P. (eds) (2000a) *What Works? Evidence-based Policy and Practice in Public Services*. Bristol: Policy Press.

Davies, H., Nutley, S. and Smith, P. (2000b) 'Introducing evidence-based policy and practice in public services', in H. Davies, S. Nutley and P. Smith (eds) *What Works: Evidence-based Policy and Practice in Public Services*. Bristol: Policy Press.

Davis, P. and Howden-Chapman, P. (1996) 'Translating research findings into health policy', *Social Science and Medicine*, 43: 865–72.

Deakin, N. and Wright, A. (eds) (1990) *Consuming Public Services*. London: Routledge.

Dearden, R. (1985) *Dealing with Inequalities in Health*. Birmingham: HSMC, University of Birmingham.

Denham, J. (1999) 'Health Action Zones in 78 million pound trailblazing "money for modernisation" Zones will lead the way in modernising services and tackling inequalities', DH Press Release 1999/0034. London: DH.

Department of Environment, Transport and the Regions (1998) *Modern Local Government: In Tough with the People*. London: DETR.

Department of Environment, Transport and the Regions (2000a) *Regeneration Research Summary: Collaboration and Co-ordination in Area-based Regeneration Initiatives*, no. 35. Online. Available http://www.dltr.gov.uk.

Department of Environment, Transport and the Regions (2000b) *Regeneration Research Summary: Measuring Multiple Deprivation at the Small Area Level: The Indices of Deprivation 2000*, no. 37. Online. Available http://www.dltr.gov.uk.

Department of Environment, Transport and the Regions (2000c) *Regeneration Research Summary: A Review of the Evidence Base for Regeneration Policy and Practice*, no. 39. Online. Available http://www.dltr.gov.uk.

Department of Environment, Transport and the Regions (2000d) *Local Strategic Partnerships*, consultation document. London: DETR.

Department of Environment, Transport and the Regions (2001) *Local Strategic Partnerships Government Guidance*. Online. Available http://www.local-regions.detr.gov.uk/lsp/guidance/index.htm.

Department of Environment, Transport and the Regions (2002) *Collaboration and Co-ordination in Area-based Regeneration Initiatives*, final report. London: DETR.

Department of Health (1989) *Caring for People: Community Care in the Next Decade and Beyond*, Cm 849. London: HMSO.

Department of Health (1991) *The Patient's Charter: Raising the Standard*. London: HMSO.

Department of Health (1995) *Variations in Health: What Can the Department of Health and NHS Do?* London: DH.

Department of Health (1997a) *Health Action Zones – Invitation to Bid*, Circular EL (97)65. Leeds: NHSE.

Department of Health (1997b) *Health Action Zones*, Circular EL (97)145. Leeds: NHSE.

Department of Health (1998a) *Evaluation of Health Action Zones: Research Brief.* London: Department of Health Research and Development Division.

Department of Health (1998b) 'Frank Dobson gives the go ahead for the first wave of Health Action Zones', Press Release 98/120. London: DH.

Department of Health (1998c) 'Fifteen new Health Action Zones to tackle health inequalities', Press Release 98/329. London: DH.

Department of Health (1998d) *Our Healthier Nation: A Contract for Health*, a consultation paper, Cm 3852. London: The Stationery Office.

Department of Health (1999a) *National Service Framework for Mental Health.* London: DH. Online. Available http://www.doh.gov.uk/nsf/.

Department of Health (1999b) *Opportunity for All: Tackling Poverty and Social Exclusion*, first annual report, Cm 4445. London: HMSO.

Department of Health (1999c) *Reducing Health Inequalities: An Action Report.* London: DH.

Department of Health (1999d) *Saving Lives: Our Healthier Nation.* London: The Stationery Office.

Department of Health (1999e) 'Seven million people to benefit from fifteen new Health Action Zones further action taken to reduce health inequalities', Press Release 99/0259. London: DH.

Department of Health (2000a) *Healthy Living Centres.* Online. Available http://www.doh.gov.uk/hlc.

Department of Health (2000b) *National Service Framework for Coronary Heart Disease.* London: DH. Online. Available http://www.doh.gov.uk/nsf/coronary1.htm.

Department of Health (2000c) *The NHS Plan.* London: The Stationery Office. Online. Available http://www.doh.gov.uk/nhsplan/default.htm.

Department of Health (2001a) *From Vision to Reality.* London: The Stationery Office.

Department of Health (2001b) *The National Health Inequalities Targets (Updated targets).* London: DH. Online. Available http://www.doh.gov.uk/healthinequalities/targets.pdf.

Department of Health (2001c) *National Service Framework for Older People.* London: The Stationery Office.

Department of Health (2001d) *Shifting the Balance of Power within the NHS.* London: The Stationery Office. Online. Available http://www.doh.gov.uk/shiftingthebalance/.

Department of Health (2001e) *Involving Patients and the Public in Health Care: A Discussion Document.* London: DH.

Department of Health (2002a) *Tackling Health Inequalities through Local Public Service Agreements.* London: Department of Health. Online. Available http://www.doh.gov.uk/lpsa/guidance-tackling-health-inequalities.htm.

Department of Health (2002b) *Tackling Health Inequalities: Summary of the 2002 Cross-cutting Review.* London: The Stationery Office.

Department of Health (2003a) *Compendium of Clinical and Health Indicators 2002.* London: The Stationery Office.

Department of Health (2003b) Letter to HAZ Project Managers: 'Health Action Zone revenue resource allocations for PCTs', 28 January. London: DH.

Department of Health (2003c) *Tackling Health Inequalities: A Programme for Action*. London: The Stationery Office. Online. Available http://www.doh.gov.uk/healthinequalities/programmeforaction/programmeforaction.pdf.

Department of Health and HM Treasury (2002) *Tackling Health Inequalities: Summary of the 2002 Cross-cutting Review*. London: DH.

Department of Health and Social Security (1975) *A Joint Approach to Social Policies*. London: HMSO.

Department of Health R&D Division (1998) *Evaluation of Health Action Zones: Research Brief*. London: Department of Health.

Dobson, F. (1997) ' "Health Action Zones" envisaged as co-operative NHS partnerships', DH Press Release 97/145. London: DH.

Donaldson, L. (2001) *Annual Report of the Chief Medical Officer to the Department of Health: On the State of the Public Health*. London: DH.

Donkin, A., Goldblatt, P. and Lynch, K. (2002) 'Inequalities in life expectancy by social class, 1972–1999', *Health Statistics Quarterly*, 15 (autumn): 5–15.

Doyle, N. (2001) 'Modernisation and public health', *Health Development Today*, 4 (July): 8.

Drever, F. and Whitehead, M. (eds.) (1997) *Health Inequalities: Decennial Supplement*. London: The Stationery Office.

Duncan, C., Jones, K. and Moon, G. (1996) 'Health-related behaviour in context: a multilevel approach', *Social Science and Medicine*, 42: 817–30.

Ellis, K. (1993) *Squaring the Circle: User and Carer Participation in Needs Assessment*. York: Joseph Rowntree Foundation.

Evans, D. (2003) 'Implementing policies to tackle health inequalities at the local level', in A. Oliver and M. Exworthy (eds) *Health Inequalities: Evidence, Policy and Implementation: Proceedings from a Meeting of the Health Equity Network*. London: The Nuffield Trust.

Evans, D. and Killoran, A. (2000) 'Tackling health inequalities through partnership working: learning from a realistic evaluation', *Critical Public Health*, 10: 125–40.

Evans, D., Mays, N. and Wyke, S. (2001) 'Evaluating complex policies: what have we learned from total purchasing?', in N. Mays, S. Wyke, G. Malbon and N. Goodwin (eds) *The Purchasing of Health Care from Primary Care Organisations*. Buckingham: Open University Press.

Exworthy, M. and Peckham, S. (1998) 'The contribution of coterminosity to joint purchasing in health and social care', *Health and Place*, 4: 233–43.

Exworthy, M., Powell, M., Berney, L. and Hallam, E. (2000) *Understanding Health Variations and Policy Variations*, Research Findings from the Health Variations Programme, Issue 5. London: ESRC Health Variations Programme.

Exworthy, M., Berney, L. and Powell, M.A. (2002) ' "How great expectations in Westminster may be dashed locally": the local implementation of national policy on health inequalities', *Policy and Politics*, 30: 79–96.

Exworthy, M., Stuart, M., Blane, D. and Marmot, M. (2003) *Tackling Health Inequalities since the Acheson Inquiry*. Bristol: Policy Press for the Joseph Rowntree Foundation.

Ferlie, E., Ashburner, L., Fitzgerald, L. and Pettigrew, A. (1996) *The New Public Management in Action*. Oxford: Oxford University Press.

Fischer, F. (2003) *Reframing Public Policy: Discursive Politics and Deliberative Practices*. Oxford: Oxford University Press.

Freeman, J. (2002) 'Mainstreaming matters', *Health Development Today*, 11 (October/November): 15–17.

Fulbright-Anderson, K., Kubisch, A.C. and Connell, J.P. (eds) (1998) *New Approaches to Evaluating Community Initiatives. Volume 2: Theory, Measurement, and Analysis*. Washington, DC: The Aspen Institute. Online. Available http://www.aspenroundtable.org/.

Fulop, N., Elston, J., Hensher, M., McKee, M. and Walters, R. (1998) 'Evaluation of the implementation of *The Health of the Nation*', *The Health of the Nation – A Policy Assessed*. London: The Stationery Office.

Geser, E. (2002) *East London Cardiovascular Health Communities Fund Programme 1999–2002: An Evaluation*. London: East London and the City HAZ.

Gesler, W. (1992) 'Therapeutic landscapes: medical issues in the light of the new cultural geography', *Social Science and Medicine*, 34: 735–46.

Geva-May, I and Pal, L. (1999) 'Good fences make good neighbours: policy evaluation and policy analysis – exploring the differences', *Evaluation*, 5: 259–77

Gilles, P. (1998) 'Effectiveness of alliances and partnerships for health promotion', *Health Promotion International*, 13: 99–120.

Glendinning, C., Powell, M. and Rummery, K. (eds) (2002) *Partnerships, New Labour and the Governance of Welfare*. Bristol: Policy Press.

Goodman, A. and Webb, S. (1994) *For Richer, for Poorer: The Changing Distribution of Income in the United Kingdom 1961–91*. London: Institute for Fiscal Studies.

Gordon, D., Shaw, M., Dorling, D. and Davey Smith, G. (eds.) (1999) *Inequalities in Health: The Evidence Presented to the Independent Inquiry into Inequalities in Health, Chaired by Sir Donald Acheson*. Bristol: Policy Press.

Gordon, D., Adelman, L., Ashworth, K., Bradshaw, J., Levitas, R., Middleton, S., Pantazis, C., Patsios, D., Payne, S., Townsend, P. and Williams, J. (2000) *Poverty and Social Exclusion in Britain*. York: Joseph Rowntree Foundation.

Goumans, M. and Springett, J. (1997) 'From projects to policy: "Healthy Cities" as a mechanism for policy change?', *Health Promotion International*, 12: 311–22.

Graham, H. (ed.) (2000a) *Understanding Health Inequalities*. Buckingham: Open University Press.

Graham, H. (2000b) 'The challenge of health inequalities', in H. Graham (ed.) *Understanding Health Inequalities*. Buckingham: Open University Press.

Graham, H. (2004) 'Tackling inequalities in health in England: remedying health disadvantage, narrowing health gaps or reducing health gradients', *Journal of Social Policy*, 33: 115–31.

Griffiths, R. (1988) *Community Care: Agenda for Action*. London: HMSO.

Guba, E. and Lincoln, Y. (1988) 'The countenances of fourth-generation evaluation: description, judgment, and negotiation', *Evaluation Studies Review Annual*, 11: 70–88.

Hadley, R. and Clough, R. (1996) *Care in Chaos*. London: Cassell.

Hall, S., Beazley, M. and associates (1996) *The Single Regeneration Budget: A Review of Challenge Fund Round II*. Birmingham: Centre for Urban and Regional Studies, the University of Birmingham.

Hampton, W. (1990) 'Planning', in N. Deakin and A. Wright (eds) *Consuming Public Services*. London: Routledge.

Hansard (2000a) 'Prime Minister's Question Time 28th June: Mr Charles Kennedy', *Hansard*, Col 901. London: House of Commons.

Hansard (2000b) 'Adjournment debate: Health Action Zones 12 July', *Hansard*, Col 179WH–199WH. London: House of Commons.

Harrison, S. (1998) 'The politics of-evidence based medicine in the United Kingdom', *Policy and Politics*, 26: 15–32.

Hattersley, L. (1999) 'Trends in life expectancy by social class – an update', *Health Statistics Quarterly*, 2: 16–24.

Health Development Agency (2003) *Tackling Health Inequalities: Turning Policy into Practice?* London: Health Development Agency.

Henry, G.T. (2002) 'Choosing criteria to judge program success', *Evaluation*, 8: 182–204.

Higgins, J. (1998) 'HAZ warnings', *Health Services Journal*, 108(5600): 24–5.

Hill, M. (1997) 'Implementation theory: yesterday's issue?', *Policy and Politics*, 25: 375–85.

Hiscock, J. and Pearson, M. (1999) 'Looking inwards, looking outwards: dismantling the "Berlin Wall" between health and social services?', *Social Policy and Administration*, 33: 150–63.

Hoskins, R. and Smith, L. (2002) 'Nurse-led welfare benefits screening in a general practice located in a deprived area', *Public Health*, 116: 214–20.

House, E. and Howe, K. (1999) *Values in Evaluation and Social Research.* Thousand Oaks, CA: Sage.

House of Commons (2002) Minutes of Evidence for Wednesday 17th October 2001: Select Committee on Public Expenditure, Examination of Witnesses: (questions 20–30) Alan Milburn MP, Jacqui Smith MP, Mr Richard Douglas, Mr Giles Denham and Mr Neil Mckay, London: House of Commons, HC281 1.

Hudson, B., Hardy, B., Henwood, M. and Wistow, G. (1999) 'In pursuit of inter-agency collaboration in the public sector: what is the contribution of theory and research?', *Public Management*, 1: 235–60.

Hughes, J., Knox, C., Murray, M. and Greer, J. (1998) *Partnership Governance in Northern Ireland: The Path to Peace.* Dublin: Oak Tree Press.

Humber Forum for Health and Regeneration (2000) *Advancing Together for Health*: 60 examples of innovative partnerships from Health Action Zones across Yorkshire and Humber. Edited by John Calaghan of Bradford Health Action Zone with support from the Department of Health.

Humpage, L. and Fleras, A. (2001) 'Intersecting discourses: closing the gaps, social justice and the treaty of Waitangi', *Social Policy Journal of New Zealand*, 16: 37–53.

Hunter, D. (2003) 'Evidence-based policy and practice: riding for a fall?', *Journal of the Royal Society of Medicine*, 96: 194–6.

Hunter, D., Warner, M., Beddow, T., Cohen, D., Connelly, J., Hardy, B., Longley, M., Richards, C., Robinson, M., Sykes, W., Taylor, D., Williams, R. and Wistow, G. (1998) 'Investing in health? An assessment of the impact of *The Health of the Nation*', *The Health of the Nation – A Policy Assessed*. London: The Stationery Office.

Huxham, C. (ed.) (1996) *Creating Collaborative Advantage.* London: Sage.

Huxham, C. and Vangen, S. (2000) 'What makes partnerships work?' in S.P. Osborne (ed) *Public–Private Partnerships: Theory and Practice in International Perspective*, London: Routledge.

Jacobs, B., Mulroy, S. and Sime, C. (2002) 'Theories of change and community involvement in North Staffordshire health action zone', in L. Bauld and K. Judge (eds) *Learning from Health Action Zones*. Chichester: Aeneas.

Jones, G.R. and George, G.M. (1998) 'The experience and evolution of trust: Implications for Cooperation and Teamwork', *Academy of Management Review*, 23: 531–46.

Jowell, T. (1999) 'Health action zones are in the frontline in the war on health inequalities: trailblazers to report to Ministers on action to drive up local standards of health', DH Press Release 1999/0038. London: DH.

Judge, K. (2000) 'Testing evaluation to the limits: the case of English Health Action Zones', *Journal of Health Services Research and Policy*, 5: 3–6.

Judge, K. and Bauld, L. (2001) 'Strong theory, flexible methods: evaluating complex, community-based initiatives', *Critical Public Health*, 11: 19–38.

Judge, K. and Mackenzie, M. (2002) 'Theory-based evaluation: new approaches to evaluating complex community-based initiatives', in J. Mackenbach and M. Bakker (eds) *Reducing Inequalities in Health: A European Perspective*. London: Routledge.

Judge, K., Barnes, M., Bauld, L., Benzeval, M., Killoran, A., Robinson, R., Wigglesworth, R. and Zeilig, H. (1999) *Health Action Zones: Learning to Make a Difference*. Canterbury: PSSRU (Personal Social Services Research Unit), University of Kent. Online. Available http://www.ukc.ac.uk/PSSRU/downloads/ddphazexec.html.

Kawachi, I., Kennedy, B. and Lochner, K. (1997) 'Long live community: social capital as public health', *The American Prospect*, Nov.–Dec.: 56–9.

Kawachi, I., Subramanian, S.V. and Almeida-Fiho, N. (2002) 'A glossary for health inequalities', *Journal of Epidemiology and Community Health*, 56: 647–52.

Killoran, A. and Popay, J. (2002) 'Concepts and methods; stakeholders perspectives of local systems for tackling health inequalities.' An exploratory study. London Health Development Agency. Available online at http://www.hda.nhs.uk/evidence.

Klein, R. (2000) 'From evidence-based medicine to evidence-based policy?', *Journal of Health Services Research & Policy*, 5: 65–6.

Klein, R. (2003) 'Commentary: making policy in a fog', in A. Oliver and M. Exworthy (eds) *Health Inequalities: Evidence, Policy and Implementation. Proceedings from a Meeting of the Health Equity Network*. London: The Nuffield Trust.

Lambeth, Southwark and Lewisham Health Action Zone (2003) 'A Big Thank You', *HAZ News*. London: LSL HAZ.

Lane, C. and Bachmann, R. (1998) *Trust Within and Between Organisations*. Oxford: Oxford University Press.

Laughlin, S. and Black, D. (1995) *Poverty and Health: Tools for Change*. Birmingham: Public Health Trust.

Ledwith, M. (1997) *Participating in Transformation. Towards a Working Model of Community Empowerment*. Birmingham: Venture Press.

LeGrand, J. and Bartlett, W. (eds) (1993) *Markets and Social Policy*. London: Macmillan.

Lindholm, L. and Rosen, M. (2000) 'What is the "gold standard" for assessing population-based interventions? Problems of dilution bias', *Journal of Epidemiology and Community Health*, 54: 617–22.

Ling, T. (2002) 'Delivering joined-up government in the UK: dimensions, issues and problems, *Public Administration*, 80: 615–42.

Local Government Association (LGA) (2000) *Partnerships with Health: A Survey of Local Authorities*. London: LGA.

Lomas, J. (2000) 'Connecting research and policy', *Canadian Journal of Policy Research*, 1: 140–4.

Luke, J.S. (1997) *Catalytic Leadership: Strategies for an Interconnected World*. New York: Jossey-Bass.

Macintyre, S. (1997a) 'The Black report and beyond what are the issues?', *Social Science and Medicine*, 44: 723–45.

Macintyre, S. (1997b) 'What are spatial effects and how can we measure them?', in A. Dale (ed.) *Exploiting National Survey Data: The Role of Locality and Spatial Effects*. Manchester: Faculty of Economic and Social Studies, University of Manchester.

Macintyre, S. (2001) 'Socio-economic inequalities in health in Scotland', in Scottish Executive (ed.) *Social Justice Annual Report 2001*. Edinburgh: Scottish Executive.

Macintyre, S. (2003a) 'Evaluating evidence on measures to reduce inequalities in health', in A. Oliver and M. Exworthy (eds) *Health Inequalities: Evidence, Policy and Implementation. Proceedings from a Meeting of the Health Equity Network*. London: The Nuffield Trust.

Macintyre, S. (2003b) 'Evidence based policy making', *British Medical Journal*, 326: 5–6.

Macintyre, S., Chalmers, I., Horton, R. and Smith, R. (2001) 'Using evidence to inform policy: a case study', *British Medical Journal*, 322: 222–5.

Macintyre, S., Ellaway, A. and Cummins, S. (2002) 'Place effects on health: how can we conceptualise, operationalise and measure them?', *Social Science and Medicine*, 55: 125–39.

Macintyre, S., McKay, L., Der, G. and Hiscock, R. (2003) 'Socio-economic position and health: what you observe depends on how you measure it', *Journal of Public Health Medicine*, 25: 288–94.

Mackenbach, J. (2003) 'Speakers Corner: Tackling inequalities in health: the need for building a systematic evidence base', *Journal of Epidemiology and Community Health*, 57: 162.

Mackenbach, J. and Bakker, M. (eds.) (2002) *Reducing Inequalities in Health: A European Perspective*. London: Routledge.

Mackenbach, J. and Kunst, A. (1997) 'Measuring the magnitude of socio-economic inequalities in health: an overview of available measures illustrated with two examples from Europe', *Social Science and Medicine*, 44: 757–71.

Mackenzie, M. (2002) *Starting Well's Theory of Change: Implications for Implementation and Evaluation*. Glasgow: Health Promotion Policy Unit, University of Glasgow.

Mackenzie, M. and Blamey, A. (2005) 'The theory and the practice: the application of a theories of change approach', *Evaluation*, 11: 193–210.

Mackenzie, M., Lawson, L., Blamey, A. and Judge, K. (2001a) *New Deal for Communities: National Evaluation – Scoping Phase, Analysis of Delivery Plans within the Health Domain*. Glasgow: Health Promotion Policy Unit, University of Glasgow.

Mackenzie, M., Lawson, L., Mackinnon, J., Meth, F. and Truman, J. (2001b) *Health Action Zones: Integrated Case Studies – Preliminary Findings.* Glasgow: Health Promotion Policy Unit, University of Glasgow.

Mackenzie, M., Lawson, L. and Mackinnon, J. (2002) 'Generating learning', in L. Bauld and K. Judge (eds) *Learning from Health Action Zones.* Chichester: Aeneas.

Mackenzie, M., Lawson, L., Mackinnon, J., Meth, F. and Truman, J. (2003) *National Evaluation of Health Action Zones. The Integrated Case Studies: A Move towards Whole Systems Change.* Glasgow: Health Promotion Policy Unit, University of Glasgow.

MacKian, S. (2002) 'Complex cultures: rereading the story about health and social capital', *Critical Social Policy,* 22: 203–25.

Mackintosh, M. (1992) 'Partnerships: issues of policy and negotiation', *Local Economy,* 7: 210–24.

McVea, J. (2003) *Demonstration Project Programme Future Strategy – Draft Framework for Action in Moving Towards a Second Phase.* Edinburgh: Scottish Executive.

Manor, O., Matthews, S. and Power, C. (1997) 'Comparing measures of health inequality', *Social Science and Medicine,* 45: 761–71.

Martin, R. (2001) 'Geography and public policy: the case of the missing agenda', *Progress in Human Geography,* 25: 189–210.

Martin, S. and Sanderson, I. (1999) 'Evaluating public policy experiments: measuring outcomes, monitoring processes or managing pilots?', *Evaluation,* 5: 245–58.

Massey, D. (2001) 'Geography on the agenda', *Progress in Human Geography,* 25: 5–17.

Mayer, R.C., Davis, J.H. and Schoorman, F.D. (1995) 'An integrative model of organizational trust', *Academy of Management Review,* 20: 709–34.

Maynard, R. (2000) 'Whether a sociologist, economist psychologist or simply a skilled evaluator: lessons from evaluation practice in the United States', *Evaluation,* 6: 471–80.

Mays, N., Goodwin, N., Malbon, G. and Wyke, S. (2001) 'Health service developments: what can be learned from the UK total purchasing experiment?', in N. Mays, S. Wyke, G. Malbon and N. Goodwin (eds) *The Purchasing of Health Care by Primary Care Organisations: An Evaluation and Guide to Future Policy.* Buckingham: Open University Press.

Milburn, A. (1997) '£30 million for new partnerships to target health inequalities', DH Press Release 97/312. London: DH.

Milligan, C. (2001) *Geographies of Caring: Space, Place and the Voluntary Sector.* Aldershot: Ashgate.

Mitchell, R., Dorling, D. and Shaw, M. (2000a) *Inequalities in Life and Death: What if Britain were More Equal?* Bristol: Policy Press.

Mitchell, R., Gleave, S., Bartley, M., Wiggins, R. and Joshi, H. (2000b) 'Do attitude and area influence health? A multilevel approach to health inequalities', *Health and Place,* 6: 67–79.

Moon, G. and Brown, T. (2000) 'Governmentality and the spatialized discourse of policy: the consolidation of the post-1989 NHS reforms', *Transactions of the Institute of British Geographers,* 25: 65–76.

Multiple Risk Factor Intervention Trial Research Group (1982) 'Multiple risk factor intervention trial: risk factor changes and mortality results', *JAMA,* 248: 1465–77.

National Evaluation of Sure Start (NESS) (2000) *National Evaluation of Sure Start: Methodology Report Executive Summary.* London: Institute for the Study of Children, Families and Social Issues, Birkbeck, University of London. Online. Available http://www.ness.bbk.ac.uk (accessed 6 August 2003).

National Institute for Epidemiology (1998) Public Health Common Dataset 1996, NIE, University of Surrey, Guildford.

Nazroo, J. (1999) 'Ethnic inequalities in health', in D. Gordon, M. Shaw, D. Dorling and G. Davey Smith (eds) *Inequalities in Health: The Evidence Presented to the Independent Inquiry into Inequalities in Health, Chaired by Sir Donald Acheson.* Bristol: The Policy Press.

New Deal for Communities (NDC) Evaluation Team (2002) *NDC National Evaluation: Responding to Findings from the Scoping Stage.* London: Neighbourhood Renewal Unit, Office of the Deputy Prime Minister, NDC Programme Note 5/2002. Online. Available http://www.neighbourhood.gov.uk/ndcprognotes.asp?pageid=91.

Newman, J. (1996) 'Beyond the vision: cultural change in the Public Sector' *Public Money and Management*, April/June: 59–64.

NHS Management Executive (1992) Local Voices: The Views of Local People in Purchasing for Health. London: NHSME.

NHSE (1996) *Priority and Planning Guidance for the NHS: 1997/98.* Leeds: NHSE.

NHSE, Institute of Health Services Management (IHSM) and NHS Confederation (1998) *In the Public Interest: Developing a Strategy for Public Participation.* Leeds: NHSE.

Nutbeam, D., Smith C., Murphy, S. and Catford, J. (1993) 'Maintaining evaluation designs in long term community-based health promotion programs: the Heartbeat Wales case study', *Journal of Epidemiological Community Health*, 47: 127–33.

Nutley, S. and Webb, J. (2000) 'Evidence and the policy process', in H. Davies, S. Nutley and P. Smith (eds) *What Works?* Bristol: Policy Press, pp. 13–41.

Nutley, S., Davies, H. and Walter, I. (2002) *Evidence Based Policy and Practice: Cross-sector Lessons from UK*, ESRC working paper. London: ESRC UK Centre for Evidence Based Policy and Practice.

Nutley, S., Walter, I. and Davies, H. (2003) 'From knowing to doing: a framework for understanding the evidence-into-practice agenda', *Evaluation* 9: 125–48.

Oliver, A. and McDaid, D. (2002) 'Evidence-based health care: benefits and barriers', *Social Policy and Society*, 1: 183–90.

ONS (2002) *Regional Trends 2002 Edition.* London: The Stationery Office. Online. Available www.statistics.gov.uk/downloads/theme_compendia/Regional_Trends_37.

Owen, J. and Rogers, P. (1999) *Program Evaluation: Forms and Approaches.* London: Sage.

Painter, C. with Clarence, E. (2001) 'UK local action zones and changing urban governance', *Urban Studies*, 38: 1215–32.

Parsons, W. (1995) *Public Policy: An Introduction to the Theory and Practice of Policy Analysis.* Cheltenham: Edward Elgar.

Patton, M.Q. (1998) *Utilization-focused Evaluation: The New Century Text.* Thousand Oaks, CA: Sage.

Pawson, R. (2003) 'Nothing as practical as a good theory', *Evaluation*, 9: 471–90.

Pawson, R. and Tilley, N. (1997) *Realistic Evaluation*. London: Sage.

Pedler, M. (1998) 'Including the excluded, a case study of action learning and whole system development in Walsall', unpublished article.

Peters, B.G. and Pierre, J. (2001) 'Developments in intergovernmental relations: towards multi-level governance', *Policy and Politics*, 29: 131–6.

Petticrew, M. and Macintyre, S. (2001) 'What do we know about the effectiveness and cost-effectiveness of measures to reduce inequalities in health?', in A. Oliver, R. Cookson and D. McDaid (eds) *The Issues Panel for Equity in Health: The Discussion Papers*. London: The Nuffield Trust.

Pettigrew, A.M., Ferlie, E. and McKee, L. (1992) *Shaping Strategic Change: Making Change in Large Organisations. The Case of the National Health Service*. London: Sage.

Phillimore, P., Beattie, A. and Townsend, P. (1994) 'Widening inequality of health in Northern England, 1981–91', *British Medical Journal*, 308: 1125–9.

Platt, S., Parry, O., Ritchie, D., Gnich, W. and Major, K. (2003) *Evaluation of a Community-based Anti-smoking Intervention in a Low Income Area: A Quasi-experimental Study*. Edinburgh: Research Unit in Health, Behaviour and Change, University of Edinburgh.

Plesk, P. and Greenhalgh, P.M. (2001) 'The challenge of complexity in health care', *British Medical Journal*, 323: 625–8.

Plesk, P. and Wilson, T. (2001) 'Complexity, leadership and management in health-care organizations', *British Medical Journal*, 323: 746–9.

Plewis, I. (1998) 'Inequalities, targets and zones', *New Economy*, 5: 104–8.

Popay, J., Williams, G., Thomas, C. and Gatrell, A. (1998) 'Theorising inequalities in health: the place of lay knowledge', in M. Bartley, D. Blane and G. Davey Smith (eds) *The Sociology of Health Inequalities*. London: Blackwell.

Popay, J., Thomas, C., Williams, G., Bennett, S., Gatrell, A. and Bostock, L. (2003) 'A proper place to live: health inequalities, agency and the normative dimensions of space', *Social Science and Medicine*, 57: 55–69.

Powell, M. (1999) 'New Labour and the third way in the British National Health service', *International Journal of Politics*, 29: 353–70.

Powell, M. and Exworthy, M. (2001) 'Joined-up solutions to address health inequalities: analysing policy, process and resource streams', *Public Money and Management*, 21: 21–6.

Powell, M. and Moon, G. (2001) 'Health Action Zones: the "third" way of a new area-based policy?', *Health and Social Care in the Community*, 9: 43–50.

Powell, M., Boyne, G. and Ashworth, R. (2001a) 'Towards a geography of people poverty and place poverty', *Policy and Politics*, 29: 243–58.

Powell, M., Exworthy, M. and Berney, L. (2001b) 'Playing the game of partner-ship', in R. Sykes, C. Bochel and N. Ellison (eds) *Social Policy Review*, 13: 39–61.

Rahman, M., Palmer, G., Kenway, P. and Howarth, C. (2000) *Monitoring Poverty and Social Exclusion 2000*. York: Joseph Rowntree Foundation.

Rathwell, T. (1992) 'Pursuing health for all in Britain – an assessment', *Social Science and Medicine*, 34: 169–82.

Rees, P., Brown, D., Norman, P. and Dorling, D. (2003) 'Are socioeconomic inequalities in mortality decreasing or increasing within some British regions? An observational study, 1990–1998', *Journal of Public Health Medicine*, 25: 208–14.

Reid, A. and Harding, S. (2000) 'Trends in regional deprivation and mortality using the Longitudinal Study', *Health Statistics Quarterly*, 5: 17–25.

Rhodes, R. (1997) *Understanding Governance: Policy Networks, Governance, Reflexivity and Accountability*. Buckingham: Open University Press.

Richards, S., Barnes, M., Coulson, A., Gaster, L., Leach, B. and Sullivan H. (1999) *Cross-Cutting Issues in Public Policy and Public Services*. London: DETR.

Rittel, H. and Webber, M. (1973) 'Dilemmas in a general theory of planning', *Policy Sciences*, 4: 155–69.

Roberts, V. and associates (1995) *Public/Private/Voluntary Partnerships in Local Authorities*. Luton: Local Government Management Board.

Robson, B., Parkinson, M., Robinson, F. and associates (1994) *Assessing the Impact of Urban Policy*. London: HMSO.

Rossi, P. and Wright, J. (1987) 'Evaluation research: an assessment', *Evaluation Studies Review Annual*, 11: 48–69.

Rousseau, D.M., Sitkin, S.B., Burt, R.S. and Camerer, C. (1998) 'Not so different after all: a cross-discipline view of trust', *Academy of Management Review*, 23: 339–404.

Rummery, K. (1998) 'Changes in primary health care policy: the implications for joint commissioning with social services', *Health and Social Care in the Community*, 6: 429–38.

Rummery, K. and Coleman, A. (2003) 'Primary care and social services in the UK: progress towards partnership?', *Social Science and Medicine*, 56: 1773–82.

Russell, H. (2001) *Local Strategic Partnerships: Lessons from the New Commitment to Regeneration*. Bristol: Policy Press.

Sanderson, I. (2000) 'Evaluation in complex policy systems', *Evaluation*, 6: 433–54.

Sanderson, I. (2001) 'Performance management, evaluation and learning in "modern" local government', *Public Administration*, 79: 297–313.

Sanderson, I. (2002) 'Evaluation, policy learning and evidence based policy making', *Public Administration*, 80: 1–22.

Savas, E.S. (2000) *Privatization and Public–Private Partnerships*. New York: Seven Bridges Press.

Schorr, L. (1998) *Learning what Works: Evaluating Complex Social Interventions*, Report on the Symposium. New York: Governmental Studies Program, The Brooking Institution.

Scriven, M. (1984) 'Evaluation ideologies', *Evaluation Studies Review Annual*, 9: 48–80.

Shaw, I. and Crompton, A. (2003) 'Theory, like mist on spectacles, obscures vision', *Evaluation*, 9: 192–204.

Shaw, M., Dorling, D., Gordon, D. and Davey Smith, G. (1999) *The Widening Gap: Health Inequalities and Policy in Britain*. Bristol: Policy Press.

Sheffield First for Health (2002) *If Only We Knew What We Know Now*. Sheffield: Sheffield First for Health.

Shouls, S., Congdon, P. and Curtis, S. (1996) 'Modelling inequality in reported long term illness in the UK: combining individual and area characteristics', *Journal of Epidemiology and Community Health*, 50: 366–76.

Sloggett, A. and Joshi, H. (1994) 'Higher mortality in deprived areas: community or personal disadvantage?', *British Medical Journal*, 309: 1470–4.

Social Exclusion Unit (1998) *Bringing Britain Together: A National Strategy for Neighbourhood Renewal*, Cm 4045. London: The Stationery Office.

Social Exclusion Unit (1999) *Teenage Pregnancies*. London: The Stationery Office.

Social Exclusion Unit (2000) *Joining it up Locally*, PAT 17 Report. London: The Stationery Office.

Social Exclusion Unit (2001) *A New Commitment to Neighbourhood Renewal, National Strategy Action Plan*. London: The Stationery Office.

Social Exclusion Unit (2004) *Tackling Social Exclusion: Taking Stock and Looking to the Future*. London: Office of the Deputy Prime Minister. Online. Available http:www.socialexclusionunit.gov.uk.

Solesbury, W. (2001) *Evidence-based Policy: Whence It Came and Where It's Going*. London: ESRC UK Centre for evidence based policy and practice, Queen Mary, University of London, ESRC UK Centre for evidence based policy and practice working paper 1, available at http://www.evidencenetwork.org/cgi-win/ enet.exe/pubs?QMV (downloaded 01 July 2003).

Sorensen, G., Emmons, K., Hunt, E.K. and Johnston. D. (1998) 'Implications of the results of community intervention trials', *Annual Review of Public Health*, 19: 379–416

SPMT (Strategic Policy Making Team) (1999) *Professional Policy Making for the Twenty-first Century*. London: Cabinet Office.

Stewart, J. and Stoker, G. (eds) (1995) *Local Government in the 1990s*. London: Macmillan.

Stewart, M., Goss, S., Gillanders, G., Clarke, R., Rowe, J. and Shaftoe, H. (1999) *Cross-cutting Issues Affecting Local Government*. London: DETR.

Stewart, M., Gillanders, G., Goss, S., Grimshaw, L., Cameron, S. and Healy, P. (2002) *Collaboration and Co-ordination in Area-based Regeneration Initiatives*, final report to the Department of Transport, Local Government and the Regions. London: DETR.

Stocking, B. (1985) *Initiative and Inertia: Case Studies in the NHS*. London: The Nuffield Provincial Hospitals Trust.

Strong, M., Maheswaran, R., Fryers, P. and White, P. (2002) 'Are socioeconomic inequalities in mortality decreasing in the Trent region UK? An observational study', *Journal of Public Health Medicine*, 24: 120–2.

Subramanian, S.V., Lochner, K. and Kawachi, I. (2003) 'Neighbourhood differences in social capital: a compositional artefact or contextual construct?', *Health and Place*, 9: 33–44.

Sullivan, H. and Skelcher, C. (2002) *Working across Boundaries: Collaboration in Public Services*. Basingstoke: Palgrave.

Sullivan, H. and Stewart, M. (2002) *'Joining-up' Governance – The Co-ordination and Integration of Arrangements in Northern Ireland*. Briefing paper for the Review of Public Administration in Northern Ireland, December. Available at: http://www.rpani.gov.uk/briefingpapers.

Sullivan, H., Smith, M. and Knight, T. (1999) *Working in Partnership: Evaluating Northumberland HAZ*. Birmingham: School of Public Policy, University of Birmingham.

Sullivan, H., Barnes, M. and Matka, E. (2002) 'Building collaborative capacity through "theories of change": early lessons from the evaluation of Health Action Zones in England', *Evaluation*, 8: 205–26.

Sullivan, H., Knops, A., Barnes, M. and Newman, J. (2003a) 'Central–local relations in an era of multi-level governance: the case of public participation policy in England, 1997–2001', submitted to *Local Government Studies*, July.

Sullivan, H., Newman, J., Barnes, M. and Knops, A. (2003b) 'The role of institutions in facilitating and constraining dialogue in partnerships with communities', in C. Scott and W.E. Thurston (eds) *Collaboration in Context*. Calgary: University of Calgary.

Sullivan, H., Judge, K. and Sewel, K. (2004) '"In the eye of the beholder": Perceptions of local impact in English Health Action Zones', *Social Science and Medicine*, 59(8): 1603–12.

Sutherland, H., Sefton, T. and Piachaud, D. (2003) Poverty in Britain: the impact of government policy since 1997. York: Joseph Rowntree Foundation.

Swann, C. and Morgan, A. (2002) *Social Capital for Health: Insights from Qualitative Research*. London: Health Development Agency.

Timmins, N. (1995) *The Five Giants: A Biography of the Welfare State*. London: HarperCollins.

Townsend, P. and Davidson, N. (1982) 'The Black Report', in P. Townsend, M. Whitehead and N. Davidson (eds) *Inequalities in Health: The Black Report and the Health Divide*, new edition, London: Penguin.

Tudor Hart, J. (1971) 'The inverse care law', *The Lancet*, 1: 405–12.

Veenstra, G. and Lomas, J. (1999) 'Home is where the governing is: social capital and regional health governance', *Health and Place*, 5: 1–12.

Verma, N. (1998) *Similarities, Connections and Systems: The Search for a New Rationality for Planning and Management*. Lanham, MD: Lexington Books.

Vernon, P., MacDermott, K., Nessling, B., Findlay, G. and Dear, S. (2002) *Investing our Learning in the Future: Key Strategic Learning from the London and Luton Health Action Zones*. London: Lambeth, Southwark and Lewisham HAZ.

Wanless, D. (2004) *Securing Good Health for the Whole Population*. London: The Stationery Office.

Weiss, C. (1995a) 'The haphazard connection: social science and public policy', *International Journal of Education Research*, 23: 137–50.

Weiss, C. (1995b) 'Nothing as practical as good theory: exploring theory-based evaluation for comprehensive community initiatives for children and families', in J. Connell, A. Kubisch, L. Schorr and C. Weiss (eds) *New Approaches to Evaluating Community Initiatives: Concepts, Methods and Contexts*. Washington, DC: The Aspen Institute.

Weiss, C. (1998) 'Have we learned anything new about the use of evaluation?', *American Journal of Evaluation*, 19: 21–33.

Weiss, C. (1998b) *Evaluation: Methods for Studying Programs and Policies* (2nd edn). Upper Saddle River, NJ: Prentice Hall.

Whitehead, M. (1992) 'The concepts and principles of equity in health', *International Journal of Health Services*, 22: 429–45.

Whitehead, M. and Drever, F. (1999) 'Narrowing social inequalities in health? Analysis of trends in mortality among babies of lone mothers', *British Medical Journal*, 318: 908–14.

Wholey, J. (1983) *Evaluation and Effective Public Management*. Boston, MA: Little, Brown.

Wiggins, R., Bartley, M., Gleave, S., Joshi, H., Lynch, K. and Mitchell, R. (1998) 'Limiting long-term illness: a question of where you live or who you are? A multi-level analysis of the 1971–1991 ONS longitudinal study', *Risk Decision and Policy*, 3: 181–98.

Wilkinson, D. (1997) 'Whole system development: rethinking public service management', *International Journal of Public Sector Management*, 19: 505–33.

Wilkinson, D. and Appelbee, E. (1999) *Implementing Holistic Government: Joined Up Action on the Ground*. Bristol: The Policy Press.

Wismar, M. and Busse, R. (2002) 'Outcome-related health targets – political strategies for better health outcomes: a conceptual and comparative study', *Health Policy*, 59: 223–41.

Yanow, D. (2003) 'Accessing local knowledge', in M.A. Hajer and H. Wagenaar (eds) *Deliberative Policy Analysis: Understanding Governance in the Network Society*. Cambridge: Cambridge University Press.

Young, I.M. (2000) *Inclusion and Democracy*. Oxford: Oxford University Press.

Index

The following abbreviations are used in the index:
HAZ = Health Action Zone
NHS = National Health Service
PCT = Primary Care Trust